POCKET GUIDE TO
NURSING DIAGNOSES

POCKET GUIDE TO

NURSING DIAGNOSES

THIRD EDITION

Mi Ja Kim, RN, PhD, FAAN
Professor, Acting Dean,
College of Nursing,
University of Illinois at Chicago,
Chicago, Illinois

Gertrude K. McFarland, RN, DNSc, FAAN
Health Scientist Administrator, Nursing Research
Study Section,
Division of Research Grants,
National Institutes of Health, USPHS,
U.S. Department of Health and Human Services,
Bethesda, Maryland

Audrey M. McLane, RN, PhD
Professor Emerita,
College of Nursing,
Marquette University,
Milwaukee, Wisconsin

The C. V. Mosby Company

St. Louis • Baltimore • Philadelphia • Toronto 1989

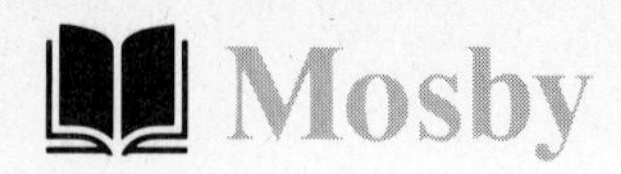

Editor: William Grayson Brottmiller
Senior developmental editor: Sally Adkisson
Project manager: Kathleen L. Teal
Production editor: Judith Bange
Design: Rey Umali

Third edition

Printed in the United States of America

The C.V. Mosby Company
11830 Westline Industrial Drive, St. Louis, Missouri 63146

Library of Congress Cataloging in Publication Data

Pocket guide to nursing diagnoses.

Bibliography: p.
Includes index.
1. Diagnosis—Handbooks, manuals, etc. 2 . Nursing—Handbooks, manuals, etc. I. Kim, Mi Ja. II. McFarland, Gertrude K. III. McLane, Audrey M.
RT48.P63 1989 616.07′5 88-33037
ISBN 0-8016-3274-9

GW/D/D 9 8 7 6 5 4 3 2 1

CONTRIBUTORS

Kim Astroth, RN, BSN

Graduate Student, Department of Adult Health Nursing, College of Nursing—Urbana Regional Site, University of Illinois, Urbana, Illinois

Thelma I. Bates, RN, MSN, CS

Psychiatric Clinical Specialist, Washington Hospital Center, Washington, D.C.

Joan M. Caley, RN, MS, CS*

Associate Chief, Nursing Service/Extended Care, Veterans Administration Medical Center, Portland, Oregon

Nancy Creason, RN, PhD

Associate Professor, Department of Medical-Surgical Nursing, College of Nursing–Urbana Regional Site, University of Illinois, Urbana, Illinois

Kathryn Czurylo, RN, MS

Surgical Clinical Nurse Specialist, Alexian Brothers Medical Center, Elk Grove, Illinois

Donna M. Dixon, BSN, MS

Doctoral Student, College of Nursing, University of Illinois at Chicago; Assistant Professor, Saint Xavier College, Chicago, Illinois

---

*The opinions expressed herein are those of the authors and do not necessarily reflect those of the National Institutes of Health, U.S. Public Health Service, U.S. Department of Health and Human Services, or the Veterans Administration.

Susan Dudas, RN, MSN

Associate Professor, Department of Medical-Surgical Nursing, College of Nursing, University of Illinois at Chicago, Chicago, Illinois

Teresa Fadden, RN, MSN

Clinical Nurse Specialist—Chronic Illness, St. Joseph's Hospital, Milwaukee, Wisconsin

Richard J. Fehring, RN, DNSc

Associate Professor, Marquette University, Milwaukee, Wisconsin

Margaret I. Fitch, RN, PhD

Director, Nursing Research and Professional Development, Toronto General Hospital, Toronto, Ontario, Canada

Michile C. Gattuso, RN, MS

Alexian Brothers Medical Center, Elk Grove, Illinois

Elizabeth Kelchner Gerety, RN, MS, CS*

Clinical Nurse Specialist, Psychiatry, Psychiatry Consultation Service, Portland Veterans Administration Medical Center, Portland, Oregon

Jane E. Graydon, RN, PhD

Associate Professor, Faculty of Nursing, University of Toronto, Toronto, Ontario, Canada

Mary V. Hanley, RN, MA

Consultant in Nursing; Formerly Coordinator and Assistant Professor, Graduate Medical-Surgical Nursing Program, Boston University, Boston, Massachusetts

Kathryn Hennessey, RN, MS, CCRN

Clinical Nurse Specialist, Alexian Brothers Medical Center, Elk Grove, Illinois

Karen Kavanaugh, BSN, MSN

Instructor and Doctoral Student, University of Illinois at Chicago, Chicago, Illinois

Mi Ja Kim, RN, PhD, FAAN

Professor, Acting Dean, College of Nursing, University of Illinois at Chicago, Chicago, Illinois

Pamela Kohlbry, RN, MSN

Camarillo, California

Candice S. Korb, RN, MSN

Formerly Pediatric Home Health Care, Jewish Social Service Agency, Rockville, Maryland

Carol Kupperberg, RN, MSN

Nursing Consultant, Home Care Program, Children's Hospital National Medical Center, Washington, D.C.

Jane Lancour, RN, MSN

Doctoral Student, University of Wisconsin—Milwaukee, Milwaukee, Wisconsin; Nurse Consultant—JML and Associates, Irvine, California

Janet L. Larson, RN, PhD

Assistant Professor, Department of Medical-Surgical Nursing, College of Nursing, University of Illinois at Chicago, Chicago, Illinois

Lorna A. Larson, RN, DNSc

Program Analyst, Quality Assurance Division, Community Mental Health Services, Washington, D.C.

Marie Maguire, RN, BSN

Graduate Student—Marquette University, Milwaukee, Wisconsin; Clinical Nurse Specialist, Lakeland Nursing Home—Walworth County, Elkhorn, Wisconsin

Mary E. Markert, RN, MN

Clinical Administrator, St. Elizabeth's Campus, D.C. Commission on Mental Health Services, Washington, D.C.

Gertrude K. McFarland, RN, DNSc, FAAN*

Health Scientist Administrator, Nursing Research Study Section, Division of Research Grants, National Institutes of Health, USPHS, U.S. Department of Health and Human Services, Bethesda, Maryland

Audrey M. McLane, RN, PhD

Professor Emerita, College of Nursing, Marquette University, Milwaukee, Wisconsin

Sarah Anne McNabb, RN, BSN

Graduate Student—Marquette University; Staff Nurse, Clinical III, St. Joseph's Hospital, Milwaukee, Wisconsin

Ruth E. McShane, RN, PhD

Robert Wood Johnson Clinical Nurse Scholar, University of Rochester School of Nursing, Rochester, New York

Judy Minton, RN, BSN

Graduate Student, Department of Adult Health Nursing, College of Nursing—Urbana Regional Site, University of Illinois, Urbana, Illinois

Victoria L. Mock, RN, DNSc

Assistant Professor, School of Nursing, Boston College, Chestnut Hill, Massachusetts

Martha M. Morris, RN, EdD

Director of Nursing, St. Louis State Hospital, St. Louis, Missouri

Charlotte E. Naschinski, RN, MS

Acting Director, Nursing Education Section, D.C. Commission on Mental Health Services, Office of Training and Standards, Washington, D.C.

Colleen M. O'Brien, RN, BSN

Graduate Student—Marquette University, Milwaukee, Wisconsin; Staff Nurse—Critical Care, Denmark, Wisconsin

Linda O'Brien-Pallas, RN, PhD

Assistant Professor, Faculty of Nursing, University of Toronto, Toronto, Ontario, Canada

Annette M. O'Connor, RN, PhD

Assistant Professor, Faculty of Health Sciences, School of Nursing, University of Ottawa, Ottawa, Ontario, Canada

Catherine Ryan, RN, MS

Clinical Nurse Specialist, Alexian Brothers Medical Center, Elk Grove, Illinois

Polly Ryan, RN, MSN

Doctoral Student, University of Wisconsin—Milwaukee, Milwaukee, Wisconsin

Patricia Saskowski, RN, BSN

Graduate Student—Marquette University; ICU Staff Nurse, St. Joseph's Hospital, Milwaukee, Wisconsin

Sheila Schilling-Olson, RN, BSN

Graduate Student—Marquette University, Milwaukee, Wisconsin; Supervisor, Internal Medicine, Skemp–Grandview–La Crosse Clinic, Ltd., La Crosse, Wisconsin

Pamela M. Schroeder, RN, MSN

Staff Nurse, Mercy Health Center; M. Div. Student, Wartburg Theological Seminary, Dubuque, Iowa

Janet F. Schulte, RN, MSN

Clinical Nurse Specialist, Infertility, Genetics, and IVF Institute, Fairfax, Virginia

Karen V. Scipio-Skinner, RN, MSN

Training Supervisor, Office of Quality Assurance, American Psychiatric Association, Washington, D.C.

Maureen E. Shekleton, RN, DNSc

Assistant Professor, Department of Medical-Surgical Nursing, College of Nursing, University of Illinois at Chicago, Chicago, Illinois

Margaret J. Stafford, RN, MSN

Clinical Specialist, Cardiovascular Nursing, Hines Veterans Administration Hospital, Hines, Illinois

Rosemarie Suhayda, RN, MSN

Assistant Professor, Department of Medical-Surgical Nursing, College of Nursing, University of Illinois at Chicago, Chicago, Illinois

Alice M. Tse, BSN, MSN

Doctoral Student, College of Nursing, University of Illinois at Chicago, Chicago, Illinois

Marilyn Wade, RN, MSN

Clinical Nurse Specialist—Rehabilitation and Neurology, Columbia Hospital, Milwaukee, Wisconsin

Evelyn L. Wasli, RN, DNSc

Unit Coordinator, Intensive Care Unit, Emergency Psychiatric Response Division, Community Mental Health Services, Washington, D.C.

Linda K. Young, RN, MSN

Instructor, School of Nursing, Milwaukee County Medical Complex, Milwaukee, Wisconsin

Definition of Nursing Diagnosis

A nursing diagnosis is a clinical judgment about an individual, family, or community that is derived through a deliberate, systematic process of data collection and analysis. It provides the basis for prescriptions for definitive therapy for which the nurse is accountable. It is expressed concisely and includes the etiology of the condition when known.

Shoemaker JK: Essential features of a nursing diagnosis. In Kim MJ, McFarland GK, and McLane AM: Classification of nursing diagnoses: proceedings of the Fifth National Conference, St Louis, 1984, The CV Mosby Co, p 109.

PREFACE

In recent years the impact of nursing diagnoses on nursing practice has been widely felt across the country and in many corners of the world. National and international responses to previous editions of this *Pocket Guide* have been positive and gratifying. We are grateful for constructive suggestions received from clinicians, students, and faculty that have contributed to the third edition of this text.

The major purposes of this *Pocket Guide* are (1) to provide an easy-to-use guide for clinicians, faculty, and students in their daily practice; (2) to stimulate critical thinking of practicing nurses; and (3) to facilitate theory and research-based nursing interventions in the practice setting.

In keeping with the philosophy of the previous editions, every effort has been made to make this *Pocket Guide* easy to use while providing a theoretical and empirical data base for each prototype care plan. We have chosen to present nursing diagnoses in alphabetical order because the conceptual framework for the organization of nursing diagnoses is still under development. The current NANDA Taxonomy I—revised version, however, uses a different organizational approach and is presented in Appendix B.

One noteworthy additional feature of this edition is a conceptual approach to assessment categories. Fifteen assessment categories were developed on the basis of content analysis of current nursing diagnoses, which were approved by NANDA at the Eighth National Conference held in 1988. These categories have taken into account the major tenets of nursing, person, health, and environment.

To facilitate the use of these categories and help nurses to remember 15 categories, the following acronym is proposed: ABC^4 PRN REST For Health. *A* stands for activity/rest, *B* for beliefs/decision making, C^1 for cardiopulmonary function, C^2

for comfort, C^3 for cognitive/perceptual factors, C^4 for communicating, *P* for physical integrity, *R* for role/relationship, *N* for nutrition, *R* for resource management, *E* for elimination, *S* for sensory/motor function, *T* for thermoregulation, *F* for feeling, and *H* for host defense function.

Defining characteristics and related/risk factors presented are NANDA approved, and the same is true for the majority of definitions. Definitions of nursing diagnoses approved by NANDA have been used to the extent they were developed. For completeness, we developed definitions for those diagnoses without definitions—rape trauma syndrome: compound reaction and rape trauma syndrome: silent reaction.

A concerted effort has been made to present nursing care plans as prototypes rather than standard care plans. By making the care plans prototypes, we have emphasized that they are for specific individuals or a group of patients with specified related factors. Therefore, in applying these plans to patients, practicing nurses will need to give specific consideration to individual patient requirements. Acuity and severity of nursing diagnoses are other dimensions that were not addressed in these care plans for the sake of brevity, but these are other important factors for nurses to consider when individualizing these care plans.

Each care plan was developed on the basis of a nursing diagnosis that comprises a diagnostic label and the term *related to* for selected related or risk factors. For example, if the nursing diagnosis is Potential for Injury with a risk factor of "emotional liability," the nurse would record this as "Potential for injury related to emotional liability." We used the following guide for the development of the prototype care plans:

1. The goal statement reflects a desired health state of a patient that results from selected nursing interventions.
2. Nursing interventions are selected in order to address related factors or risk factors, to ameliorate defining characteristics, to assist patients in achieving their goals, and to attain an optimal health state.
3. Expected outcomes address the extent of achievement of patient goals, evaluate the effectiveness of nursing interventions, and include modification of defining characteristics of a nursing diagnosis.

The care plans were developed from a holistic perspective of persons interacting with their environment in the pursuit of health. Contributing authors of this *Pocket Guide* are clinical experts who reflect the state of the art of nursing practice. References provided for each care plan have been updated to communicate the most current theory and/or research bases for proposed nursing interventions.

The use of nursing diagnoses to generate interventions has sharpened the focus on current practice and has demonstrated the potential of these diagnoses for contributing to quality health care. We acknowledge substantive contributions made by practicing nurses to the development and refinement of nursing diagnoses. Practicing nurses are encouraged to engage in critical thinking while using the prototype care plans. Their participation in research on missing diagnoses is essential for the national and international development of nursing diagnoses taxonomy and a scientific base for nursing practice.

Mi Ja Kim
Gertrude K. McFarland
Audrey M. McLane

CONTENTS

ASSESSMENT CATEGORIES

Pattern recognition, validating judgments, and interpretation of meaning within a particular context are basic cognitive skills registered nurses bring to a pätient/family health care situation. Pattern recognition in response to cues (defining characteristics) may occur at any point in the assessment process. Assessment data may be gathered to facilitate pattern recognition and/or to validate the existence of a previously recognized pattern.

Subjective and objective assessment data are gathered with respect to the presenting situation or longer-term health status, activities and demands of daily living, and internal and external resources (current and potential) of the patient/family (Carnevali, 1983). Nursing diagnoses, agreed-on labels for the diagnostic concepts, are assigned to the patterns recognized. A nursing diagnosis for a patient/family health care situation includes a diagnostic label and related factors contributing to the onset or maintenance of the diagnosis. Validation and interpretation of the diagnosis and related factors are ongoing processes of cue and pattern recognition. A nursing diagnosis, then, becomes the focal point for developing goals, expected outcomes, and interventions.

To facilitate the assessment process, nursing diagnoses are broadly categorized in the areas of psychosocial human functioning and physiological regulation. We developed the following acronym, ABC^4 PRN REST For Health, in order to help nurses remember the assessment categories, which include nursing diagnoses, in their daily practice:

A Activity/rest
B Beliefs/decision making

C[1] Cardiopulmonary (breathing/circulation)
C[2] Comfort
C[3] Cognitive/perceptual (perception/cognition)
C[4] Communicating (communication)

P Physical integrity
R Role/relationship
N Nutrition

R Resource management
E Elimination
S Sensory/motor
T Thermoregulation

F Feeling
H Host defense

Nursing diagnoses under each of these assessment categories are listed in Appendix A.

Activity/rest

The activity/rest category includes patterns that are self-selected by individuals in response to biological clocks and/or imposed by demands or limitations of disease or illness. Activity/rest patterns evolve in response to available energy and energy expenditures required to engage in daily personal care activities, work, exercise, and leisure. Energy is made available through a normal pattern of nutrition, breathing, circulation, and sufficient rest/sleep to support a desired pattern of human activity. Physical disabilities may place limits on activities or may require excess expenditures of energy to engage in daily personal care activities.

Beliefs/decision making

The beliefs/decision making category includes patterns of response to the selection of a treatment alternative, following a prescribed therapeutic regimen, and/or a personal decision to achieve a health goal. Beliefs/decision making can be altered by challenges to values, history of previous health care decisions, methods of coping with stress, and spiritual well-being.

Cardiopulmonary

The cardiopulmonary category includes patterns of circulation and gas exchange. The cardiopulmonary function can be altered by tracheobronchial infection; decreased energy/fatigue; excessive airway secretions; perceptual/cognitive impairment; dysfunctional swallowing mechanisms to prevent aspiration; pain; neuromuscular impairment; severe anxiety; alterations in mechanical, electrical, and structural functions of the heart; hemorrhage; excessive intake of sodium and fluid; or interruption in arterial or venous flow.

Comfort

The comfort category includes patterns of acute and chronic pain. Pain responses are influenced by the nature of stressor(s), psychological state, and cultural and societal norms. Patterns of response to pain evolve and/or are learned as individuals are exposed to their own pain and the pain of significant others. Responses to pain can be altered by the person's pain history, methods used to cope with pain, and the family/significant other's response to the person in pain. An expectation that discomfort will increase with disease progression is an important factor.

Cognitive/perceptual

The cognitive/perceptual category includes patterns of cognitive operations, activities, and knowledge acquisition, as well as perceptions about the various aspects of sex. Cognitive operations and activities, such as memory, decision making, problem solving, learning, orientation, and reality-based thinking, evolve over time as an individual develops and are influenced by learning taking place within the context of the family, community, and culture. Life occurrences, such as physiological changes and physical illness, or psychological conflicts and psychiatric illness, can impact on normal patterns and result in memory loss, impaired judgment, distractibility, and decreased ability to learn. The individual's self-concept includes that person's perception of his/her own capabilities, self-worth, identity, and body image. Psychosocial and cultural factors play an important role in shaping a person's own perception of self.

Communicating

The communicating category includes patterns of verbal communication influenced by an individual's physical and emotional conditions and developmental state. Communication patterns are learned within a family and cultural context. Physical barriers, such as brain tumors, or anatomic deficits can result in impaired articulation or the inability to find words and name objects. Psychiatric conditions can lead to such manifestations as flight of ideas, incessant verbalization, or loose association of ideas. Cultural differences may create difficulties for the individual in speaking the dominant language. To understand communication patterns, the originator of the message (sender), the means of sending the message, the recipient of the message (receiver), and the feedback provided by the receiver must be taken into account.

Physical integrity

The physical integrity category includes patterns of optimal physical status. Physical integrity can be altered by reduced vision and/or olfactory sensation, occupational hazards, an adverse environment, impaired motor abilities, dehydration, trauma, noxious agents, malnutrition, infection, decreased salivation, altered circulation, hyperthermia or hypothermia, chemical substance, radiation, or immobilization.

Role/relationship

The role/relationship category describes patterns of role relationships and responsibilities, such as family/parenting roles, sexuality patterns, and social roles. A well-functioning family enables the growing and developing child to experience nurturing others in an environment that fosters optimal growth. Situational or developmental transition or crises, however, can result in family dysfunction and result in an inability of the family system to meet the physical, emotional, and spiritual needs of its members. The absence of supportive family, friends, and meaningful groups can be experienced as a sense of aloneness or social isolation. Any one of a number of factors can lead to impaired social interaction—insufficient knowledge about ways to enhance mutuality, impaired communication, poor self-esteem, limited mobility, sociocultural dissonance, and limited life interests. The role/relationship category also includes sexuality, or the behavioral expression of a person's sexual identity. It includes, but is not limited to, sexual relationships with a partner.

Nutrition

The nutrition category includes patterns of nutritional intake that are self-selected by individuals in response to the psychological state, cultural and societal norms, the presence of a normal gastrointestinal tract, and/or demands or limitations of disease or illness. Food preferences are subject to available food supplies and resources, which places restrictions on personal and family goals influenced by nutrition. Surgical procedures may alter the gastrointestinal tract temporarily or permanently and lead to altered patterns of nutrition.

Resource management

The resource management category includes patterns of home maintenance management that evolve in response to resources available, formal and informal learning, family and community support systems, and the level of wellness or degree of illness of the individual, family, and significant others. Difficulties experienced by family members in maintaining their home in a comfortable and safe fashion are important considerations. This can include inadequate financial resources for needed repairs or assistance in cleaning.

Elimination

The elimination category includes patterns that evolve in response to an individual's perception of a normal pattern of elimination, the availability of toileting facilities, the availability of fiber-rich foods, ingestion of fluids, and the use of laxatives/enemas/suppositories to establish a desired pattern of elimination. Physical disabilities, especially those precipitated by neuromuscular diseases and spinal cord injuries, produce major changes in the complex mechanisms required for a normal pattern of elimination. Surgical procedures and the use of indwelling catheters place individuals at risk of becoming incontinent.

Sensory/motor

The sensory/motor category includes patterns of afferent and efferent neural responses. The sensory/motor function can be altered by abnormal sympathetic response to noxious stimuli, pain, perceptual/cognitive impairment, neuromuscular impairment, musculoskeletal impairment, depression/severe anxiety, inactivity, excessive environmental stimuli, electrolyte imbalance, psychological stress, mechanical obstruction (tracheotomy tube, tumor, edema, etc.), an irritated oropharyngeal cavity, hemianopsia, neurological illness, or trauma.

Thermoregulation

The thermoregulation category includes patterns of altered body temperature. Body temperature can be altered by several factors, including adverse environments, dehydration, extreme activities, altered metabolic rate, sedation, illness, or trauma affecting temperature regulation.

Feeling

The feeling category includes patterns of mood and emotions, such as anxiety, fear, grieving, hopelessness, powerlessness, post-trauma response, and potential violence. Emotions are related to a number of complex interrelated factors, including, but not limited to, unconscious conflicts, unmet needs, environmental demands, internal and external stressors, biochemical and physiological changes, learned behavior, social network, and role models. Depending on their severity, emotions can impede constructive daily functioning and, if severe, can lead to suicide or homicide.

Host defense

The host defense category includes patterns of infection and any other clinical problems that result from altered function of the immune system. The body's host defense mechanism can be altered by inadequate primary and/or secondary defenses, immunosuppressive agents, inadequate acquired immunity, chronic disease, environmental hazards, invasive procedures, malnutrition, or trauma.

BIBLIOGRAPHY

Carnevali DL: Nursing care planning: diagnosis and management, ed 3, Philadelphia, 1983, JB Lippincott Co.

Gordon M: Nursing diagnosis: process and application, ed 2, St Louis, 1987, The CV Mosby Co.

Kim MJ, McFarland GK, and McLane AM, eds: Classification of nursing diagnoses: proceedings of the Fifth National Conference, St Louis, 1984, The CV Mosby Co.

Kim MJ and Moritz DA, eds: Classification of nursing diagnoses: proceedings of the Third and Fourth National Conferences, St Louis, 1982, McGraw-Hill Book Co.

SECTION ONE

Nursing diagnoses: definitions, related/risk factors, and defining characteristics

Activity intolerance

■ **Definition** The state in which an individual has insufficient physiological or psychological energy to endure or complete required or desired daily activities.

Related factors

Generalized weakness
Sedentary life-style
Imbalance between oxygen supply and demand
Bed rest or immobility

Defining characteristics

Verbal report of fatigue or weakness
Abnormal heart rate or blood pressure response to activity
Exertional discomfort or dyspnea
Electrocardiographic changes reflecting arrhythmias or ischemia

Activity intolerance, potential

■ **Definition** The state in which an individual is at risk of experiencing insufficient physiological or psychological energy to endure or complete required or desired daily activities.

Risk factors

History of previous intolerance
Deconditioned status
Presence of circulatory/respiratory problems
Inexperience with the activity

Adjustment, impaired

■ **Definition** The state in which an individual is unable to modify his/her life-style/behavior in a manner consistent with a change in health status.

Related factors

Disability requiring change in life-style

Inadequate support systems
Impaired cognition
Sensory overload
Assault to self-esteem
Altered locus of control
Incomplete grieving

Defining characteristics

Verbalization of nonacceptance of health status change
Nonexistent or unsuccessful ability to be involved in problem solving or goal setting
Lack of movement toward independence
Extended period of shock, disbelief, or anger regarding health status change
Lack of future-oriented thinking

Airway clearance, ineffective

■ **Definition** The state in which an individual is unable to clear secretions or obstructions from the respiratory tract to maintain airway patency.

Related factors

Decreased energy and fatigue
Tracheobronchial
  Infection
  Obstruction
  Secretion
Perceptual/cognitive impairment
Trauma

Defining characteristics

Abnormal breath sounds—rales (crackles), rhonchi (wheezes)
Changes in rate or depth of respiration
Tachypnea
Cough, effective or ineffective, with or without sputum
Cyanosis
Dyspnea
Fever

Anxiety

■ **Definition** A vague, uneasy feeling, the source of which is often nonspecific or unknown to the individual.

Related factors

Unconscious conflict about essential values and goals of life
Threat to self-concept
Threat of death
Threat to or change in health status
Threat to or change in socioeconomic status
Threat to or change in role functioning
Threat to or change in environment
Threat to or change in interaction patterns
Situational and maturational crises
Interpersonal transmission and contagion
Unmet needs

Defining characteristics

Subjective
- Increased tension
- Apprehension
- Increased helplessness
- Uncertainty
- Fearful
- Scared
- Feelings of inadequacy
- Shakiness
- Fear of unspecific consequences
- Regretful
- Overexcited
- Rattled
- Distressed
- Jittery

Objective
- Sympathetic stimulation—cardiovascular excitation, superficial vasoconstriction, pupil dilation
- Restlessness
- Insomnia
- Glancing about

Poor eye contact
Trembling; hand tremors
Extraneous movements—foot shuffling; hand, arm movements
Expressed concern regarding changes in life events
Worried
Anxious
Facial tension
Voice quivering
Focus on self
Increased wariness
Increased perspiration

Aspiration, potential for

■ **Definition** The state in which an individual is at risk for entry of gastric secretions, oropharyngeal secretions, or exogenous food or fluids into tracheobronchial passages due to dysfunction or absence of normal protective mechanisms.

Risk factors

Reduced level of consciousness
Depressed cough and gag reflexes
Presence of tracheotomy or endotracheal tube
Overinflated tracheotomy/endotracheal tube cuff
Inadequate tracheotomy/endotracheal tube cuff inflation
Gastrointestinal tubes
Bolus tube feedings/medication administration
Situations hindering elevation of upper body
Increased intragastric pressure
Increased gastric residual
Decreased gastrointestinal motility
Delaying gastric emptying
Impaired swallowing
Facial/oral/neck surgery or trauma
Wired jaws

Body image disturbance

■ **Definition** Disruption in the way one perceives one's body image.

Related factors

Biophysical
Cognitive perceptual
Psychosocial
Cultural or spiritual

Defining characteristics

Either the following A or B must be present to justify the diagnosis of body image disturbance:

A. Verbal response to actual or perceived change in structure and/or function

B. Nonverbal response to actual or perceived change in structure and/or function

The following clinical manifestations may be used to validate the presence of A or B:

Objective

Missing body part
Actual change in structure and/or function
Not looking at body part
Not touching body part
Hiding or overexposing body part (intentional or unintentional)
Trauma to nonfunctioning part
Change in social involvement
Negative feelings about body
Feelings of helplessness, hopelessness, or powerlessness

Preoccupation with change or loss
Emphasis on remaining strengths, heightened achievement
Extension of body boundary to incorporate environmental objects
Personalization of part or loss by name
Depersonalization of part or loss by impersonal pronouns
Refusal to verify actual change

It may be possible to identify high-risk populations such as those with the following conditions:

Missing parts

Dependence on machine
Significance of body part or functioning with regard to age, sex, developmental level, or basic human needs
Physical change caused by biochemical agents (drugs)
Physical trauma or mutilation
Pregnancy and/or maturational changes

Body temperature, altered, potential

■ **Definition** The state in which an individual is at risk for failure to maintain body temperature within normal range.

Risk factors

Extremes of age
Extremes of weight
Exposure to cold/cool or warm/hot environments
Dehydration
Inactivity or vigorous activity
Medications causing vasoconstriction/vasodilation, altered metabolic rate, sedation
Inappropriate clothing for environmental temperature
Illness or trauma affecting temperature regulation

Bowel elimination, altered

See Bowel incontinence; Constipation; Constipation, colonic; Constipation, perceived; Diarrhea.

Bowel incontinence

■ **Definition** The state in which an individual experiences a change in normal bowel habits characterized by involuntary passage of stool.

Related factors

Neuromuscular involvement
Musculoskeletal involvement
Depression; severe anxiety
Perception or cognitive impairment

Defining characteristic

Involuntary passage of stool

Breastfeeding, ineffective

■ **Definition** The state in which a mother, infant, and/or family experiences dissatisfaction or difficulty with the breastfeeding process.

Related factors

Prematurity
Infant anomaly
Maternal breast anomaly
Previous breast surgery
Previous history of breastfeeding failure
Infant receiving supplemental feedings with artificial nipple
Poor infant sucking reflex
Nonsupportive partner/family
Knowledge deficit
Interruption in breastfeeding

Defining characteristics

Unsatisfactory breastfeeding process
Actual or perceived inadequate milk supply
Infant's inability to attach on to maternal nipple correctly
No observable signs of oxytocin release
Observable signs of inadequate infant intake
Nonsustained suckling at breast
Suckling at only one breast per feeding
Nursing less than 7 times in 24 hours
Persistence of sore nipples beyond first week of life
Maternal reluctance to put infant to breast as necessary
Infant exhibiting fussiness and crying within first hour after breastfeeding; unresponsive to other comfort measures
Infant arching and crying at breast; resisting latching on

Breathing pattern, ineffective

■ **Definition** The state in which an individual's inhalation and/or exhalation pattern does not enable adequate ventilation.

Related factors
Neuromuscular impairment
Pain
Musculoskeletal impairment
Perception or cognitive impairment
Anxiety
Decreased energy and fatigue
Inflammatory process
Decreased lung expansion
Tracheobronchial obstruction

Defining characteristics
Dyspnea
Shortness of breath
Tachypnea
Fremitus
Abnormal arterial blood gas
Cyanosis
Cough
Nasal flaring
Respiratory depth changes
Assumption of three-point position
Pursed-lip breathing and prolonged expiratory phase
Increased anteroposterior diameter
Use of accessory muscles
Altered chest excursion

Cardiac output, decreased

■ **Definition** The state in which the blood pumped by an individual's heart is sufficiently reduced that it is inadequate to meet the needs of the body's tissues.

Related factors
Mechanical
Alteration in preload
Alteration in afterload
Alteration in inotropic changes in heart
Electrical
Alteration in rate

Alteration in rhythm
Alteration in conduction
Structural

Defining characteristics

Variations in hemodynamic readings
Arrhythmias; ECG changes
Fatigue
Jugular vein distention
Cyanosis; pallor of skin and mucous membranes
Oliguria, anuria
Decreased peripheral pulses
Cold, clammy skin
Rales
Dyspnea

Comfort, altered

See Pain; Pain, chronic.

Communication, impaired verbal

- **Definition** The state in which an individual experiences a decreased or absent ability to use or understand language in human interaction.

Related factors

Decrease in circulation to brain
Physical barrier, brain tumor, tracheostomy, intubation
Anatomic deficit, cleft palate
Psychological barriers, psychosis, lack of stimuli
Cultural difference
Developmental or age-related

Defining characteristics

Unable to speak dominant language
Does not or cannot speak
Stuttering; slurring
Impaired articulation
Dyspnea
Disorientation

Inability to modulate speech
Inability to find words
Inability to name words
Inability to identify objects
Loose association of ideas
Flight of ideas
Incessant verbalization
Difficulty with phonation
Inability to speak in sentences

Constipation

■ **Definition** The state in which an individual experiences a change in normal bowel habits characterized by a decrease in frequency and/or passage of hard, dry stools.

Related factors

Less than adequate intake
Less than adequate dietary intake and bulk
Less than adequate physical activity or immobility
Personal habits
Medications
Chronic use of medication and enemas
Gastrointestinal obstructive lesions
Neuromuscular impairment
Musculoskeletal impairment
Pain on defecation
Diagnostic procedures
Lack of privacy
Weak abdominal musculature
Pregnancy
Emotional status

Defining characteristics

Frequency less than usual pattern
Hard-formed stool
Palpable mass
Reported feeling of rectal fullness
Straining at stool
Decreased bowel sounds

Reported feeling of abdominal or rectal fullness or pressure
Less than usual amount of stool
Nausea

Other possible defining characteristics

Abdominal pain
Back pain
Headache
Interference with daily living
Use of laxatives
Decreased appetite
Appetite impairment

Constipation, colonic

- **Definition** The state in which an individual's pattern of elimination is characterized by hard, dry stool that results from a delay in passage of food residue.

Related factors

Less than adequate fluid intake
Less than adequate dietary intake
Less than adequate fiber
Less than adequate physical activity
Immobility
Lack of privacy
Emotional disturbances
Chronic use of medication and enemas
Stress
Change in daily routine
Metabolic problems (e.g., hypothyroidism, hypocalcemia, hypokalemia)

Defining characteristics

Decreased frequency
Hard, dry stool
Straining at stool
Painful defecation
Abdominal distention
Palpable mass
Rectal pressure

Headache, appetite impairment
Abdominal pain

Constipation, perceived

■ **Definition** The state in which an individual makes a self-diagnosis of constipation and ensures a daily bowel movement through use of laxatives, enemas, and suppositories.

Related factors

Cultural/family health beliefs
Faulty appraisal
Impaired thought processes

Defining characteristics

Expectation of a daily bowel movement with resulting overuse of laxatives, enemas, and suppositories
Expected passage of stool at same time every day

Coping, defensive

■ **Definition** The state in which an individual experiences falsely positive self-evaluation based on a self-protective pattern that defends against underlying perceived threats to positive self-regard.

Related factors

To be developed

Defining characteristics

Denial (of obvious problems/weaknesses)
Projection (of blame/responsibility)
Rationalizes failures
Defensiveness (hypersensitive to criticism)
Grandiosity
Superior attitude toward others
Difficulty establishing/maintaining relationships
Hostile laughter or ridicule of others
Difficulty in reality testing of perceptions
Lack of follow-through or participation in treatment or therapy

Coping, family: potential for growth

- **Definition** Effective managing of adaptive tasks by family member involved with the client's health challenge, who now is exhibiting desire and readiness for enhanced health and growth in regard to self and in relation to the client.

Related factors

Family members attempt to describe growth impact of crisis on their own values, priorities, goals, or relationships.

Family member is moving in direction of health-promoting and enriching life-style that supports and monitors maturational processes, audits and negotiates treatment programs, and generally chooses experiences that optimize wellness.

Individual expresses interest in making contact on a one-to-one basis or on a mutual-aid group basis with another person who has experienced a similar situation.

Coping, ineffective family: compromised

- **Definition** Insufficient, ineffective, or compromised support, comfort, assistance, or encouragement usually by a supportive primary person (family member or close friend); client may need it to manage or master adaptive tasks related to his/her health challenge.

Related factors

Inadequate or incorrect information or understanding by a primary person

Temporary preoccupation by a significant person who is trying to manage emotional conflicts and personal suffering and is unable to perceive or act effectively in regard to client's needs.

Temporary family disorganization and role changes

Other situational or developmental crises or situations the significant person may be facing

Client providing little support in turn for the primary person

Prolonged disease or disability progression that exhausts supportive capacity of significant people

Defining characteristics

Subjective

Client expresses or confirms concern/complaint about significant other's response to client's health problem

Significant person describes preoccupation with personal reactions (e.g., fear, anticipatory grief, guilt, anxiety) regarding client's illness or disability or to other situational or developmental crises

Significant person describes or confirms an inadequate understanding or knowledge base that interferes with effective assistive or supportive behaviors

Objective

Significant person attempts assistive or supportive behaviors with less than satisfactory results

Significant person withdraws or enters into limited or temporary personal communication with client at time of need

Significant person displays protective behavior disproportionate (too little or too much) to client's abilities or need for autonomy

Coping, ineffective family: disabling

■ **Definition** Behavior of significant person (family member or other primary person) that disables his/her own capacities and the client's capacities to effectively address tasks essential to either person'a adaptation to the health challenge.

Related factors

Significant person with chronically unexpressed feelings of guilt, anxiety, hostility, despair, etc.

Dissonant discrepancy of coping styles being used to deal with adaptive tasks by the significant person and client or among significant people

Highly ambivalent family relationships

Arbitrary handling of family's resistance to treatment that tends to solidify defensiveness, as it fails to deal adequately with underlying anxiety.

Defining characteristics

Neglectful care of client in regard to basic human needs and/or illness treatment

Distortion of reality regarding client's health problem, including extreme denial about its existence or severity
Intolerance
Rejection
Abandonment
Desertion
Carrying on usual routines; disregarding client's needs
Psychosomatic tendency
Taking on illness signs of client
Decisions and actions by family that are detrimental to economic or social well-being
Agitation, depression, aggression, hostility
Impaired restructuring of a meaningful life for self; impaired individualization; prolonged overconcern for client
Neglectful relationships with other family members
Client's development of helpless, inactive dependence

Coping, ineffective individual

■ **Definition** Impairment of adaptive behaviors and problem-solving abilities of a person in meeting life's demands and roles.

Related factors

Situational crises
Maturational crises
Personal vulnerability
Multiple life changes
No vacations
Inadequate relaxation
Inadequate support systems
Little or no exercise
Poor nutrition
Unmet expectations
Work overload
Too many deadlines
Unrealistic perceptions
Inadequate coping method

Defining characteristics

Verbalization of inability to cope or inability to ask for help
Inability to meet role expectations
Inability to meet basic needs
Inability to problem solve
Alteration in societal participation
Destructive behavior toward self or others
Inappropriate use of defense mechanisms
Change in usual communication patterns
Verbal manipulation
High illness rate
High rate of accidents
Overeating
Lack of appetite
Excessive smoking
Excessive drinking
Overuse of prescribed tranquilizers
Alcohol proneness
High blood pressure
Chronic fatigue
Insomnia
Muscular tension
Ulcers
Frequent headaches
Frequent neckaches
Irritable bowel
Chronic worry
General irritability
Poor self-esteem
Chronic anxiety
Emotional tension
Chronic depression

Decisional conflict (specify)

■ **Definition** A state of uncertainty about the course of action to be taken when choice among competing actions involves risk, loss, or challenge to personal life values. (Specify focus of conflict, e.g., choices regarding health, family relationships, career, finances, or other life events.)

Related factors

Unclear personal values/beliefs
Perceived threat to value system
Lack of experience or interference with decision making
Lack of relevant information
Support system deficit

Defining characteristics

Verbalized feeling of distress related to uncertainty about choices
Verbalization of undesired consequences of alternative actions being considered
Vacillation between alternative choices
Delayed decision making
Self-focusing
Physical signs of distress or tension (increased heart rate, increased muscle tension, restlessness, etc.)
Questioning personal values and beliefs while attempting to make a decision

Denial, ineffective

■ **Definition** A conscious or unconscious attempt to disavow the knowledge or meaning of an event to reduce anxiety/fear to the detriment of health.

Related factors

To be developed

Defining characteristics

Delays seeking or refuses medical attention to the detriment of health
Does not perceive personal relevance of symptoms or danger
Uses home remedies (self-treatment) to relieve symptoms
Does not admit fear of death or invalidism
Minimizes symptoms
Displaces source of symptoms to other organs

Unable to admit impact of disease on life pattern
Makes dismissive gestures or comments when speaking of distressing events
Displaces fear of impact of condition
Displays inappropriate affect

Diarrhea

■ **Definition** The state in which an individual experiences a change in normal bowel habits characterized by the frequent passage of loose, fluid, unformed stools.

Related factors

Stress and anxiety
Dietary intake
Medications
Inflammation, irritation, or malabsorption of bowel
Toxins
Contaminants
Radiation

Defining characteristics

Abdominal pain
Cramping
Increased frequency
Increased frequency of bowel sounds
Loose, liquid stools
Urgency
Changes in color

Disuse syndrome, potential for

■ **Definition** The state in which an individual is at risk for deterioration of body systems as the result of prescribed or unavoidable inactivity.

Risk factors

Paralysis
Mechanical immobilization
Prescribed immobilization

Severe pain
Altered level of consciousness

Diversional activity deficit

■ **Definition** The state in which an individual experiences a decreased stimulation from or interest or engagement in recreational or leisure activities.

Related factors

Environmental lack of diversional activity
Long-term hospitalization
Frequent, lengthy treatments

Defining characteristics

Boredom
Desire for something to do, to read, etc.
Usual hobbies cannot be undertaken in hospital

Dysreflexia

■ **Definition** The state in which an individual with a spinal cord injury at T7 or above experiences or is at risk of experiencing a life-threatening uninhibited sympathetic response of the nervous system to a noxious stimulus.

Related factors

To be developed

Defining characteristics

Individual with spinal cord injury (T7 or above) with the following:
- Paroxysmal hypertension (sudden periodic elevated blood pressure where systolic pressure is over 140 mm Hg and diastolic pressure is above 90 mm Hg)
- Bradycardia or tachycardia (pulse rate of less than 60 or over 100 beats per minute)
- Diaphoresis (above injury)
- Red splotches on skin (above injury)
- Pallor (below injury)

Headache (diffuse pain in different portions of head and not confined to any nerve distribution area)
Chilling (shivering accompanied by sensation of coldness or pallor of skin)
Conjunctival congestion (excessive amount of blood/tissue fluid in conjunctivae)
Horner's syndrome (contraction of pupil, partial ptosis of eyelid, enophthalmos, and sometimes loss of sweating over affected side of face due to paralysis of cervical sympathetic nerve trunk)
Paresthesia (abnormal sensation such as numbness, prickling, or tingling; increased sensitivity)
Pilomotor reflex (gooseflesh formation when skin is cooled)
Blurred vision
Chest pain
Metallic taste in mouth
Nasal congestion

Family processes, altered

■ **Definition** The state in which a family that normally functions effectively experiences a dysfunction.

Related factors

Situational transition and/or crises
Developmental transition and/or crises

Defining characteristics*

Family system unable to meet physical needs of its members
Family system unable to meet emotional needs of its members
Family system unable to meet spiritual needs of its members
Parents do not demonstrate respect for each other's views on child-rearing practices

*The first 13 defining characteristics are specifically from Otto H: Criteria for assessing family strengths, Fam Process 2:329-338, Sept 1963.

Inability to express or accept wide range of feelings
Inability to express or accept feelings of members
Family unable to meet security needs of its members
Inability of family members to relate to each other for mutual growth and maturation
Family uninvolved in community activities
Inability to accept or receive help appropriately
Rigidity in function and roles
Family does not demonstrate respect for individuality and autonomy of its members
Family unable to adapt to change or to deal with traumatic experience constructively
Family fails to accomplish current or past developmental task
Ineffective family decision-making process
Failure to send and receive clear messages
Inappropriate boundary maintenance
Inappropriate or poorly communicated family rules, rituals, symbols
Unexamined family myths
Inappropriate level and direction of energy

Fatigue

■ **Definition** An overwhelming sense of exhaustion and decreased capacity for physical and mental work regardless of adequate sleep.

Related factors

Overwhelming psychological or emotional demands
Increased energy requirements to perform activities of daily living
Excessive social/role demands
States of discomfort
Decreased metabolic energy production
Altered body chemistry (e.g., medications, drug withdrawal)

Defining characteristics

Verbalization of fatigue/lack of energy

Inability to maintain usual routines
Perceived need for additional energy to accomplish routine tasks
Increase in physical complaints
Emotionally labile or irritable
Impaired ability to concentrate
Decreased performance
Lethargic or listless
Disinterest in surroundings/introspection
Decreased libido
Accident prone

Fear

■ **Definition** Feeling of dread related to an identifiable source that the person validates.

Related factors

Natural or innate origins—sudden noise, loss of physical support, height, pain
Learned response—conditioning, modeling from or identification with others
Separation from support system in a potentially threatening situation (hospitalization, treatments, etc.)
Knowledge deficit or unfamiliarity
Language barrier
Sensory impairment
Phobic stimulus or phobia
Environmental stimuli

Defining characteristics

Subjective
- Increased tension
- Apprehension
- Impulsiveness
- Decreased self-assurance
- Afraid
- Scared
- Terrified
- Panic

Frightened
Jittery
Objective
Increased alertness
Concentration on source
Wide-eyed
Attack behavior
Focus on "it, out there"
Fight behavior—aggressive
Flight behavior—withdrawal
Sympathetic stimulation—cardiovascular excitation, superficial vasoconstriction, pupil dilation

Fluid volume deficit (I)

■ **Definition** The state in which an individual experiences vascular, cellular, or intracellular dehydration related to failure of regulatory mechanisms.

Related factor
Failure of regulatory mechanisms
Defining characteristics
Dilute urine
Increased urine output
Sudden weight loss
Other possible defining characteristics
Possible weight gain
Hypotension
Decreased venous filling
Increased pulse rate
Decreased skin turgor
Decreased pulse volume and pressure
Increased body temperature
Dry skin
Dry mucous membranes
Hemoconcentration
Weakness
Edema
Thirst

Fluid volume deficit (2)

■ **Definition** The state in which an individual experiences vascular, cellular, or intracellular dehydration related to active loss.

Related factor

Active loss

Defining characteristics

Decreased urine output
Concentrated urine
Output greater than intake
Sudden weight loss
Decreased venous filling
Hemoconcentration
Increased serum sodium

Other possible defining characteristics

Hypotension
Thirst
Increased pulse rate
Decreased skin turgor
Decreased pulse volume and pressure
Change in mental state
Increased body temperature
Dry skin
Dry mucous membranes
Weakness

Fluid volume deficit, potential

■ **Definition** The state in which an individual is at risk of experiencing vascular, cellular, or intracellular dehydration.

Risk factors

Extremes of age
Extremes of weight
Excessive losses through normal routes (e.g., diarrhea)
Loss of fluid through abnormal routes (e.g., indwelling tubes)
Deviations affecting access to, intake of, or absorption of fluids (e.g., physical immobility)

Factors influencing fluid needs (e.g., hypermetabolic states)
Knowledge deficiency related to fluid volume
Medications (e.g., diuretics)
Increased fluid output
Urinary frequency
Thirst
Altered intake

Fluid volume excess

■ **Definition** The state in which an individual experiences increased fluid retention and edema.

Related factors

Compromised regulatory mechanism
Excessive fluid intake
Excessive sodium intake

Defining characteristics

Edema
Effusion
Anasarca
Weight gain
Shortness of breath, orthopnea
Intake greater than output
Third heart sound
Pulmonary congestion on x-ray film
Abnormal breath sounds: crackles (rales)
Change in respiratory pattern
Change in mental status
Decreased hemoglobin, hematocrit
Blood pressure changes
Central venous pressure changes
Pulmonary artery pressure changes
Jugular venous distention
Positive hepatojugular reflex
Oliguria
Specific gravity changes
Azoturia

Altered electrolytes
Restlessness and anxiety

Gas exchange, impaired

- **Definition** The state in which an individual experiences an imbalance between oxygen uptake and carbon dioxide elimination at the alveolar-capillary membrane gas exchange area.

Related factors

Altered oxygen supply
Alveolar-capillary membrane changes
Altered blood flow
Altered oxygen-carrying capacity of blood

Defining characteristics

Confusion
Somnolence
Restlessness
Irritability
Inability to move secretions
Hypercapnea
Hypoxia

Grieving, anticipatory

- **Definition** The state in which an individual grieves before an actual loss.

Related factors

Perceived potential loss of significant other
Perceived potential loss of physiopsychosocial well-being
Perceived potential loss of personal possessions

Defining characteristics

Potential loss of significant object
Expression of distress at potential loss
Denial of potential loss
Guilt
Anger

Sorrow
Choked feelings
Changes in eating habits
Alterations in sleep patterns
Alterations in activity level
Altered libido
Altered communication patterns

Grieving, dysfunctional

■ **Definition** The state in which actual or perceived object loss (object loss is used in the broadest sense) exists. Objects include people, possessions, a job, status, home, ideals, parts and processes of the body, etc.

Related factors

Actual or perceived object loss
Thwarted grieving response to a loss
Absence of anticipatory grieving
Chronic fatal illness
Lack of resolution of previous grieving response
Loss of significant others
Loss of physiopsychosocial well-being
Loss of personal possessions

Defining characteristics

Verbal expression of distress at loss
Denial of loss
Expression of guilt
Expression of unresolved issues
Anger
Sadness
Crying
Difficulty in expressing loss
Alterations in
- Eating habits
- Sleep patterns
- Dream patterns
- Activity level
- Libido

Idealization of lost object
Reliving of past experiences
Interference with life functioning
Developmental regression
Labile effect
Alterations in concentration and/or pursuits of tasks

Growth and development, altered

Definition The state in which an individual demonstrates deviations in norms from his/her age group.

Related factors

Inadequate caretaking: indifference, inconsistent responsiveness, multiple caretakers
Separation from significant others
Environmental and stimulation deficiencies
Effects of physical disability
Prescribed dependence

Defining characteristics

Delay or difficulty in performing skills (motor, social, or expressive) typical of age group
Altered physical growth
Inability to perform self-care or self-control activities appropriate for age
Flat affect
Listlessness, decreased responses

Health maintenance, altered

Definition Inability to identify, manage, and/or seek out help to maintain health.

Related factors

Lack of or significant alteration in communication skills (written, verbal, and/or gestural)
Lack of ability to make deliberate and thoughtful judgments
Perceptual or cognitive impairment
Complete or partial lack of gross and/or fine motor skills

Ineffective individual coping; dysfunctional grieving
Lack of material resources
Unachieved developmental tasks
Ineffective family coping; disabling spiritual distress

Defining characteristics

Demonstrated lack of knowledge regarding basic health practices
Demonstrated lack of adaptive behaviors to internal or external environmental changes
Reported or observed inability to take responsibility for meeting basic health practices in any or all functional pattern areas
History of lack of health-seeking behavior
Expressed interest in improving health behaviors
Reported or observed lack of equipment, financial, and/or other resources
Reported or observed impairment of personal support system

Health-seeking behaviors (specify)

■ **Definition** The state in which a client in stable health is actively seeking ways to alter personal health habits and/or the environment in order to move toward optimal health. (*Stable health status* is defined as age-appropriate illness prevention measures achieved; the client reports good or excellent health, and signs and symptoms of disease, if present, are controlled.)

Related factors

To be developed

Defining characteristics

Expressed or observed desire to seek higher level of wellness
Stated or observed unfamiliarity with wellness community resources
Demonstrated or observed lack of knowledge in health promotion behaviors

Expressed or observed desire for increased control of health practice
Expression of concern about effects of current environmental conditions on health status

Home maintenance management, impaired

■ **Definition** Inability to independently maintain a safe growth-promoting immediate environment.

Related factors
Disease or injury of individual or family member
Insufficient family organization or planning
Insufficient finances
Unfamiliarity with neighborhood resources
Impaired cognitive or emotional functioning
Lack of knowledge
Lack of role modeling
Inadequate support systems

Defining characteristics
Subjective
Household members express difficulty in maintaining their home in a comfortable fashion
Household requests assistance with home maintenance
Household members describe outstanding debts or financial crises
Objective
Disorderly surroundings
Unwashed or unavailable cooking equipment, clothes, or linen
Accumulation of dirt, food wastes, or hygienic wastes
Offensive odors
Inappropriate household temperature
Overtaxed family members (e.g., exhausted, anxious family members)
Lack of necessary equipment or aids
Presence of vermin or rodents
Repeated hygienic disorders, infestations, or infections

Hopelessness

■ **Definition** The subjective state in which an individual sees limited or no alternatives or personal choices available and is unable to mobilize energy on own behalf.

Related factors

Prolonged activity restriction creating isolation
Failing or deteriorating physiological condition
Long-term stress
Abandonment
Loss of belief in transcendent values/God

Defining characteristics

Passivity, decreased verbalization
Decreased affect
Verbal cues (indicating despondency, "I can't," sighing)
Lack of initiative
Decreased response to stimuli
Turning away from speaker
Closing eyes
Shrugging in response to speaker
Decreased appetite, increased/decreased sleep
Lack of involvement in care; passively allowing care

Hyperthermia

■ **Definition** The state in which an individual's body temperature is elevated above his/her normal range.

Related factors

Exposure to hot environment
Vigorous activity
Medications/anesthesia
Inappropriate clothing
Increased metabolic rate
Illness or trauma
Dehydration
Inability or decreased ability to perspire

Defining characteristics

Increase in body temperature above normal range
Flushed skin
Warm to touch
Increased respiratory rate
Tachycardia
Seizures/convulsions

Hypothermia*

■ **Definition** The state in which an individual's body temperature is reduced below his/her normal range but not below 35.6° C (rectal)/36.4° C (rectal, newborn).

Related factors

Exposure to cool or cold environment
Illness or trauma
Inability or decreased ability to shiver
Malnutrition
Inadequate clothing
Consumption of alcohol
Medications causing vasodilation
Evaporation from skin in cool environment
Decreased metabolic rate
Inactivity
Aging

Defining characteristics

Shivering (mild)
Cool skin
Pallor (moderate)
Slow capillary refill
Tachycardia
Cyanotic nail beds
Hypertension
Piloerection

*This diagnostic category has been revised in response to a validation study.

Incontinence, bowel

See Bowel incontinence.

Incontinence, functional

■ **Definition** The state in which an individual experiences an involuntary, unpredictable passage of urine.

Related factors

Altered environment

Sensory, cognitive, or mobility deficits

Defining characteristics

Urge to void or bladder contractions sufficiently strong to result in loss of urine before reaching an appropriate receptacle

Incontinence, reflex

■ **Definition** The state in which an individual experiences an involuntary loss of urine occurring at somewhat predictable intervals when a specific bladder volume is reached.

Related factor

Neurological impairment (e.g., spinal cord lesion that interferes with conduction of cerebral messages above level of reflex arc)

Defining characteristics

No awareness of bladder filling

No urge to void or feelings of bladder fullness

Uninhibited bladder contraction/spasm at regular intervals

Incontinence, stress

■ **Definition** The state in which an individual experiences a loss of urine of less than 50 ml occurring with increased abdominal pressure.

Related factors

- Degenerative changes in pelvic muscles and structural supports associated with increased age
- High intraabdominal pressure (e.g., obesity, gravid uterus)
- Incompetent bladder outlet
- Overdistention between voidings
- Weak pelvic muscles and structural supports

Defining characteristics

- Reported or observed dribbling with increased abdominal pressure
- Urinary urgency
- Urinary frequency (more often than every 2 hours)

Incontinence, total

■ **Definition** The state in which an individual experiences a continuous and unpredictable loss of urine.

Related factors

- Neuropathy preventing transmission of reflex indicating bladder fullness
- Neurological dysfunction causing triggering of micturition at unpredictable times
- Independent contraction of detrusor reflex due to surgery
- Trauma or disease affecting spinal cord nerves
- Anatomic (fistula)

Defining characteristics

- Constant flow of urine occurs at unpredictable times without distention or uninhibited bladder contractions/spasms
- Unsuccessful incontinence refractory to treatments
- Nocturia
- Lack of perineal or bladder-filling awareness
- Unawareness of incontinence

Incontinence, urge

■ **Definition** The state in which an individual experiences involuntary passage of urine occurring soon after a strong sense of urgency to void.

Related factors

Decreased bladder capacity (e.g., history of PID, abdominal surgeries, indwelling urinary catheter)
Irritation of bladder stretch receptors, causing spasm (e.g., bladder infection)
Alcohol
Caffeine
Increased fluids
Increased urine concentration
Overdistention of bladder

Defining characteristics

Urinary urgency
Frequency (voiding more often than every 2 hours)
Bladder contracture/spasm
Nocturia (more than 2 times per night)
Voiding in small (less than 100 ml) or in large amounts (more than 550 ml)
Inability to reach toilet in time

Infection, potential for

■ **Definition** The state in which an individual is at increased risk for being invaded by pathogenic organisms.

Risk factors

Inadequate primary defenses (broken skin, traumatized tissue, decrease in ciliary action, stasis of body fluids, change in pH secretions, altered peristalsis)
Inadequate secondary defenses (e.g., decreased hemoglobin, leukopenia, suppressed inflammatory response, immunosuppression)
Inadequate acquired immunity
Tissue destruction and increased environmental exposure
Chronic disease
Invasive procedures
Malnutrition
Pharmaceutical agents and trauma
Rupture of amniotic membranes
Insufficient knowledge to avoid exposure to pathogens

Injury, potential for

See also Poisoning, potential for; Suffocation, potential for; Trauma, potential for

■ **Definition** The state in which an individual is at risk of injury as a result of environmental conditions interacting with the individual's adaptive and defensive resources.

Risk factors

- Interactive conditions between individual and environment that impose a risk to defensive and adaptive resources of individual
- Internal
  - Biochemical
    - Regulatory function
      - Sensory dysfunction
      - Integrative dysfunction
      - Effector dysfunction
    - Tissue hypoxia
    - Malnutrition
    - Immune-autoimmune
    - Abnormal blood profile
      - Leukocytosis or leukopenia
      - Altered clotting factors
      - Thrombocytopenia
      - Sickle cell
      - Thalassemia
      - Decreased hemoglobin
  - Physical
    - Broken skin
    - Altered mobility
  - Developmental
    - Age
      - Physiological
      - Psychosocial
  - Psychological
    - Affective
    - Orientation

External
- Biological
  - Immunization level of community
  - Microorganism
- Chemical
  - Pollutants
  - Poisons
  - Drugs
    - Pharmaceutical agents
    - Alcohol
    - Caffeine
    - Nicotine
  - Preservatives
  - Cosmetics and dyes
  - Nutrients (vitamins, food types)
- Physical
  - Design, structure, and arrangement of community, building, and/or equipment
  - Mode of transport/transportation
  - Nosocomial agents
- People-provider
  - Nosocomial agents
  - Staffing patterns
  - Cognitive, affective, and psychomotor factors

Knowledge deficit (specify)

■ **Definition** The state in which specific information is lacking.

Related factors
- Lack of exposure
- Lack of recall
- Information misinterpretation
- Cognitive limitation
- Lack of interest in learning
- Unfamiliarity with information resources
- Patient's request for no information

Defining characteristics
- Verbalization of the problem

Inaccurate follow-through of instruction
Inadequate performance of test
Inappropriate or exaggerated behaviors (e.g., hysterical, hostile, agitated, apathetic)
Statement of misconception
Request for information

Mobility, impaired physical

■ **Definition** The state in which an individual experiences a limitation of ability for independent physical movement.

Related factors

Intolerance to activity; decreased strength and endurance
Pain and discomfort
Perceptual or cognitive impairment
Neuromuscular impairment
Musculoskeletal impairment
Depression; severe anxiety

Defining characteristics

Inability to purposefully move within physical environment, including bed mobility, transfer, and ambulation
Reluctance to attempt movement
Limited range of motion
Decreased muscle strength, control, and/or mass
Imposed restrictions of movement, including mechanical; medical protocol
Impaired coordination

Noncompliance (specify)

■ **Definition** A person's informed decision not to adhere to a therapeutic recommendation.

Related factors

Patient's value system
Health beliefs

Cultural influences
Spiritual values
Client and provider relationships

Defining characteristics

Behavior indicative of failure to adhere by direct observation or statements by patient or significant others
Objective tests (physiological measures, detection of markers)
Evidence of development of complications
Evidence of exacerbation of symptoms
Failure to keep appointments
Failure to progress
Inability to set or attain mutual goals

Nutrition, altered: less than body requirements

■ **Definition** The state in which an individual experiences an intake of nutrients insufficient to meet metabolic needs.

Related factor

Inability to ingest or digest food or absorb nutrients because of biological, psychological, or economic factors

Defining characteristics

Loss of weight with adequate food intake
Body weight 20% or more under ideal for height and frame
Reported inadequate food intake less than Recommended Daily Allowance
Weakness of muscles required for swallowing or mastication
Reported or evidence of lack of food
Lack of interest in food
Perceived inability to ingest food
Aversion to eating
Reported altered taste sensation
Satiety immediately after ingesting food
Abdominal pain with or without pathological conditions
Sore, inflamed buccal cavity

Nutrition, altered: more than body requirements

■ **Definition** The state in which an individual is experiencing an intake of nutrients that exceeds metabolic needs.

Related factor

Excessive intake in relationship to metabolic need

Defining characteristics

- Weight 10% over ideal for height and frame
- Weight 20% over ideal for height and frame
- Triceps skin fold greater than 15 mm in men and 25 mm in women
- Sedentary activity level
- Reported or observed dysfunctional eating patterns
  - Pairing food with other activities
  - Concentrating food intake at end of day
  - Eating in response to external cues (e.g., time of day, social situation)
  - Eating in response to internal cues other than hunger (e.g., anxiety)

Nutrition, altered: potential for more than body requirements

■ **Definition** The state in which an individual is at risk of experiencing an intake of nutrients that exceeds metabolic needs.

Risk factors

- Hereditary predisposition
- Excessive energy intake during late gestational life, early infancy, and adolescence
- Frequent, closely spaced pregnancies
- Dysfunctional psychological conditioning in relationship to food
- Membership in lower socioeconomic group
- Reported or observed obesity in one or both parents

Rapid transition across growth percentiles in infants or children
Reported use of solid food as major food source before 5 months of age
Observed use of food as reward or comfort measure
Reported or observed higher baseline weight at beginning of each pregnancy
Dysfunctional eating patterns
 Pairing food with other activities
 Concentrating food intake at end of day
 Eating in response to external cues (e.g., time of day or social situation)
 Eating in response to internal cues other than hunger (e.g., anxiety)

Oral mucous membrane, altered

■ **Definition** The state in which an individual experiences disruptions in the tissue layers of the oral cavity.

Related factors

Pathologic conditions—oral cavity (radiation to head and/or neck)
Dehydration
Trauma
 Chemical (e.g., acidic foods, drugs, noxious agents, alcohol)
 Mechanical (e.g., ill-fitting dentures; braces; tubes—endotracheal, nasogastric; surgery in oral cavity)
NPO instructions for more than 24 hours
Ineffective oral hygiene
Mouth breathing
Malnutrition
Infection
Lack of or decreased salivation
Medication

Defining characteristics

Coated tongue
Xerostomia (dry mouth)

Stomatitis
Oral lesions or ulcers
Lack of or decreased salivation
Leukoplakia
Edema
Hyperemia
Oral plaque
Oral pain or discomfort
Desquamation
Vesicles
Hemorrhagic gingivitis
Carious teeth
Halitosis

Pain

■ **Definition** The state in which an individual experiences and reports the presence of severe discomfort or an uncomfortable sensation.

Related factors

Injuring agents
- Biological
- Chemical
- Physical
- Psychological

Defining characteristics

Subjective
- Communication (verbal or coded) of pain descriptors

Objective
- Guarding behavior; protective
- Self-focusing
- Narrowed focus (altered time perception, withdrawal from social contact, impaired thought process)
- Distraction behavior (moaning, crying, pacing, seeking out other people and/or activities, restlessness)
- Facial mask of pain (eyes lack luster, "beaten look," fixed or scattered movement, grimace)
- Alteration in muscle tone (may span from listless to rigid)

Autonomic responses not seen in chronic, stable pain (diaphoresis, blood pressure and pulse rate change, pupillary dilation, increased or decreased respiratory rate)

Pain, chronic

■ **Definition** The state in which an individual experiences pain that continues for more than 6 months.

Related factor

Chronic physical/psychosocial disability

Defining characteristics

Verbal report or observed evidence of pain experienced for more than 6 months
Fear of reinjury
Physical and social withdrawal
Altered ability to continue previous activities
Anorexia
Weight changes
Changes in sleep patterns
Facial masks
Guarded movement

Parental role conflict

■ **Definition** The state in which a parent experiences role confusion and conflict in response to a crisis.

Related factors

Separation from child due to chronic illness
Intimidation with invasive or restrictive modalities (e.g., isolation, intubation)
Specialized care centers, policies
Home care of a child with special needs (e.g., apnea monitoring, postural drainage, hyperalimentation)
Change in marital status
Interruptions of family life due to home care regimen (treatments, caregivers, lack of respite)

Defining characteristics

Parent(s) expresses concerns/feelings of inadequacy to provide for child's physical and emotional needs during hospitalization or in home

Demonstrated disruption in caretaking routines

Parent(s) expresses concerns about changes in parental role, family functioning, family communication, and/or family health

Expresses concern about perceived loss of control over decisions relating to child

Reluctant to participate in normal caretaking activities even with encouragement and support

Verbalizes/demonstrates feelings of guilt, anger, fear, anxiety, and/or frustrations about effect of child's illness on family process

Parenting, altered
Parenting, altered, potential

■ **Definition** The state in which the ability of nurturing figure(s) to create an environment that promotes the optimum growth and development of another human being is altered or at risk.

Related/risk factors

Lack of available role model

Ineffective role model

Physical and psychosocial abuse of nurturing figure

Lack of support between or from significant other(s)

Unmet social and emotional maturation needs of parenting figures

Interruption in bonding process (i.e., maternal, paternal, other)

Perceived threat to own survival: physical and emotional

Mental and/or physical illness

Presence of stress: financial or legal problems, recent crisis, cultural move

Lack of knowledge

Limited cognitive functioning

- Lack of role identity
- Lack of appropriate response of child to relationship
- Multiple pregnancies
- Unrealistic expectation of self, infant, partner

Defining characteristics

- Actual and potential
  - Lack of parental attachment behaviors
    - Inappropriate visual, tactile, auditory stimulation
    - Negative identification of characteristics of infant/child
    - Negative attachment of meanings to characteristics of infant/child
  - Constant verbalization of disappointment in gender or physical characteristics of infant/child
  - Verbalization of resentment toward infant/child
  - Verbalization of role inadequacy
  - Inattention to needs of infant/child
  - Verbal disgust at body functions of infant/child
  - Noncompliance with health appointments for self and/or infant/child
  - Inappropriate caretaking behaviors (toilet training, sleep and rest, feeding)
  - Inappropriate or inconsistent discipline practices
  - Frequent accidents
  - Frequent illness
  - Growth and development lag in child
  - History of child abuse or abandonment by primary caretaker
  - Verbalizes desire to have child call parent by first name despite traditional cultural tendencies
  - Child receives care from multiple caretakers without consideration for needs of child
  - Compulsive seeking of role approval from others
- Actual
  - Abandonment
  - Runaway
  - Verbalization of inability to control child
  - Evidence of physical and psychological trauma

Personal identity disturbance

■ **Definition** Inability to distinguish between self and nonself.

Related factors
To be developed

Defining characteristics
To be developed

Poisoning, potential for

■ **Definition** Accentuated risk of accidental exposure to or ingestion of drugs or dangerous products in doses sufficient to cause poisoning.

Risk factors

- Internal (individual) factors
  - Reduced vision
  - Verbalization of occupational setting without adequate safeguards
  - Lack of safety or drug education
  - Lack of proper precaution
  - Cognitive or emotional difficulties
  - Insufficient finances
- External (environmental) factors
  - Large supplies of drugs in house
  - Medicines stored in unlocked cabinets accessible to children or confused persons
  - Dangerous products placed or stored within reach of children or confused persons
  - Availability of illicit drugs potentially contaminated by poisonous additives
  - Flaking, peeling paint or plaster in presence of young children
  - Chemical contamination of food and water
  - Unprotected contact with heavy metals or chemicals
  - Paint, lacquer, etc., in poorly ventilated areas or without effective protection
  - Presence of poisonous vegetation
  - Presence of atmospheric pollutants

Post-trauma response

- **Definition** The state in which an individual experiences a sustained painful response to (an) overwhelming traumatic event(s).

Related factors

Disaster
War
Epidemic
Rape
Assault
Torture
Catastrophic illness
Accident

Defining characteristics

Reexperience of traumatic event, which may be identified in cognitive, affective, and/or sensory motor activities (flashbacks, intrusive thoughts, repetitive dreams or nightmares, excessive verbalization of traumatic event, verbalization of survival guilt or guilt about behavior required for survival)

Psychic/emotional numbness (impaired interpretation of reality, confusion, dissociation or amnesia, vagueness about traumatic event, constricted affect)

Altered life-style (self-destructiveness such as substance abuse, suicide attempt, or other acting-out behavior; difficulty with interpersonal relationships; development of phobia regarding trauma; poor impulse control/irritability; explosiveness)

Powerlessness

- **Definition** Perception that one's own action will not significantly affect an outcome; a perceived lack of control over a current situation or immediate happening.

Related factors

Health care environment
Interpersonal interaction

Illness-related regimen
Life-style of helplessness

Defining characteristics

Severe
- Verbal expressions of having no control or influence over situation
- Verbal expressions of having no control or influence over outcome
- Verbal expressions of having no control over self-care
- Depression over physical deterioration that occurs despite patient compliance with regimens
- Apathy

Moderate
- Nonparticipation in care or decision making when opportunities are provided
- Expressions of dissatisfaction and frustration over inability to perform previous tasks and/or activities
- Does not monitor progress
- Expression of doubt regarding role performance
- Reluctance to express true feelings, fearing alienation from caregivers
- Inability to seek information regarding care
- Dependence on others that may result in irritability, resentment, anger, and guilt
- Does not defend self-care practices when challenged

Low
- Passivity
- Expressions of uncertainty about fluctuating energy levels

Rape-trauma syndrome

■ **Definition** Forced, violent sexual penetration against the victim's will and consent. The trauma syndrome that develops from this attack or attempted attack includes an acute phase or disorganization of the victim's life-style and a long-term process of reorganization of life-style.

Related factors

Inadequate support systems

Spouse-family blaming
Fear of reprisal, pregnancy, going out alone
Anxiety about potential health problems (e.g., AIDS, venereal disease, herpes)

Defining characteristics

Acute phase
- Emotional reactions
  - Anger
  - Embarrassment
  - Fear of physical violence and death
  - Humiliation
  - Revenge
  - Self-blame
- Multiple physical symptoms
- Gastrointestinal irritability
- Genitourinary discomfort
- Muscle tension
- Sleep pattern disturbance

Long-term phase
- Changes in life-style (changes in residence; dealing with repetitive nightmares and phobias; seeking family support; seeking social network support)

Rape-trauma syndrome: compound reaction

■ **Definition** An acute stress reaction to a rape or attempted rape, experienced along with other major stressors, that can include reactivation of symptoms of a previous condition.*

Related factors

Drug or alcohol abuse
History of and/or current psychiatric illness
History of and/or current physical illness

Defining characteristics

All defining characteristics listed under Rape-trauma syndrome

---

*Definition developed by Kim, McFarland, and McLane.

Reactivated symptoms of such previous conditions (i.e., physical illness, psychiatric illness)
Reliance on alcohol and/or drugs

Rape-trauma syndrome: silent reaction

■ **Definition** A complex stress reaction to a rape in which an individual is unable to describe or discuss the rape.*

Related factors

Fear of retaliation
Intense shame
Excessive denial
Lack of support

Defining characteristics

Abrupt changes in relationships with men
Increase in nightmares
Increasing anxiety during interview (e.g., blocking of associations, long periods of silence, minor stuttering, physical distress)
Marked changes in sexual behavior
No verbalization of occurrence of the rape
Sudden onset of phobic reactions

Role performance, altered

■ **Definition** Disruption in the way one perceives one's role performance.

Related factors

To be developed

Defining characteristics

Change in self-perception of role
Denial of role
Change in others' perception of role
Conflict in roles
Change in physical capacity to resume role

*Definition developed by Kim, McFarland, and McLane.

Lack of knowledge of role
Change in usual patterns or responsibility

Self-care deficit, bathing/hygiene

■ **Definition** The state in which an individual experiences an impaired ability to perform or complete bathing/hygiene activities for oneself.

Related factors
To be developed

Defining characteristics
Inability to wash body or body parts
Inability to obtain or get to water source
Inability to regulate temperature or flow

Self-care deficit, dressing/grooming

■ **Definition** The state in which an individual experiences an impaired ability to perform or complete dressing and grooming activities for onself.

Related factors
To be developed

Defining characteristics
Impaired ability to put on or take off necessary items of clothing
Impaired ability to obtain or replace articles of clothing
Impaired ability to fasten clothing
Inability to maintain appearance at satisfactory level

Self-care deficit, feeding

■ **Definition** The state in which an individual experiences an impaired ability to perform or complete feeding activities for oneself.

Related factors
To be developed

Defining characteristic
Inability to bring food from receptacle to mouth

Self-care deficit, toileting

■ **Definition** The state in which an individual experiences an impaired ability to perform or complete toileting activities for oneself.

Related factors
Impaired transfer ability
Impaired mobility status
Intolerance to activity; decreased strength and endurance
Pain, discomfort
Perceptual or cognitive impairment
Neuromuscular impairment
Musculoskeletal impairment
Depression, severe anxiety

Defining characteristics
Unable to get to toilet or commode
Unable to sit on or rise from toilet or commode
Unable to manipulate clothing for toileting
Unable to carry out proper toilet hygiene
Unable to flush toilet or empty commode

Self-concept, disturbance in

See Body image disturbance; Personal identity disturbance; Self-esteem disturbance.

Self-esteem disturbance

■ **Definition** Negative self-evaluation/feelings about self or self-capabilities, which may be directly or indirectly expressed.

Related factors
To be developed

Defining characteristics
Self-negating verbalization

Expressions of shame/guilt
Evaluates self as unable to deal with events
Rationalizes away/rejects positive feedback and exaggerates negative feedback about self
Hesitant to try new things/situations
Denial of problems obvious to others
Projection of blame/responsibility for problems
Rationalizes personal failures
Hypersensitive to criticism
Grandiosity

Self-esteem, chronic low

■ **Definition** Long-standing negative self-evaluation/feelings about self or self-capabilities.

Related factors
To be developed

Defining characteristics
Self-negating verbalization
Expressions of shame/guilt
Evaluates self as unable to deal with events
Rationalizes away/rejects positive feedback and exaggerates negative feedback about self
Hesitant to try new things/situations
Frequent lack of success in work or other life events
Overly conforming; dependent on others' opinions
Lack of eye contact
Nonassertive/passive
Indecisive
Excessively seeks reassurance

Self-esteem, situational low

■ **Definition** Negative self-evaluation/feelings about self that develop in response to a loss or change in an individual who previously had a positive self-evaluation.

Related factors
To be developed

Defining characteristics

Episodic occurrence of negative self-appraisal in response to life events in a person with a previous positive self-evaluation

Verbalization of negative feelings about self (helplessness, uselessness)

Self-negating verbalizations

Expressions of shame/guilt

Evaluates self as unable to handle situations/events

Difficulty making decisions

Sensory/perceptual alterations (specify) (visual, auditory, kinesthetic, gustatory, tactile, olfactory)

■ **Definition** The state in which an individual experiences a change in the amount or patterning of incoming stimuli accompanied by a diminished, exaggerated, distorted, or impaired response to such stimuli.

Related factors

Environmental factors

- Therapeutically restricted environments (isolation, intensive care, bed rest, traction, confining illnesses, incubator)
- Socially restricted environment (institutionalization, home-bound, aging, chronic illness, dying, infant deprivation); stigmatized (mentally ill, mentally retarded, mentally handicapped); bereaved

Altered sensory reception, transmission, and/or integration

- Neurological disease, trauma, or deficit
- Altered status of sense organs
- Inability to communicate, understand, speak, or respond
- Sleep deprivation
- Pain

Chemical alteration

- Endogenous (electrolyte imbalance, elevated BUN, elevated ammonia, hypoxia)

Exogenous (central nervous system stimulants or depressants, mind-altering drugs)
Psychological stress (narrowed perceptual fields caused by anxiety)

Defining characteristics

Disoriented in time, in place, or with persons
Altered abstraction
Altered conceptualization
Change in problem-solving abilities
Reported or measured change in sensory acuity
Change in behavior pattern
Anxiety
Apathy
Change in usual response to stimuli
Indication of body image alteration
Restlessness
Irritability
Altered communication patterns
Disorientation
Lack of concentration
Daydreaming
Hallucinations
Noncompliance
Fear
Depression
Rapid mood swings
Anger
Exaggerated emotional responses
Poor concentration
Disordered thought sequencing
Bizarre thinking
Visual and auditory distortions
Motor incoordination

Other possible defining characteristics

Complaints of fatigue
Alteration in posture
Change in muscular tension
Inappropriate responses
Hallucinations

Sexual dysfunction

- **Definition** The state in which an individual experiences a change in sexual function that is viewed as unsatisfying, unrewarding, or inadequate.

Related factors

Biopsychosocial alteration of sexuality
- Ineffectual or absent role models
- Physical abuse
- Psychosocial abuse (e.g., harmful relationships)
- Vulnerability
- Misinformation or lack of knowledge
- Values conflict
- Lack of privacy
- Lack of significant other
- Altered body structure or function: pregnancy, recent childbirth, drugs, surgery, anomalies, disease process, trauma, radiation

Defining characteristics
- Verbalization of problem
- Alterations in achieving perceived sex role
- Actual or perceived limitation imposed by disease and/or therapy
- Conflicts involving values
- Alterations in achieving sexual satisfaction
- Inability to achieve desired satisfaction
- Seeking of confirmation of desirability
- Alteration in relationship with significant other
- Change in interest in self and others

Sexuality patterns, altered

- **Definition** The state in which an individual expresses concern regarding his/her sexuality.

Related factors

Knowledge/skill deficit about alternative responses to

health-related transitions, altered body function or structure, illness, or medical treatment
Lack of privacy
Lack of significant other
Ineffective or absent role models
Conflicts with sexual orientation or variant preferences
Fear of pregnancy or of acquiring sexually transmitted disease
Impaired relationship with significant other

Defining characteristic

Reported difficulties, limitations, or changes in sexual behaviors or activities

Skin integrity, impaired

■ **Definition** The state in which an individual's skin is adversely altered.

Related factors

- External (environmental)
  - Hyperthermia or hypothermia
  - Chemical substance
  - Mechanical factors
    - Shearing forces
    - Pressure
    - Restraint
  - Radiation
  - Physical immobilization
  - Humidity
- Internal (somatic)
  - Medication
  - Altered nutritional state: obesity, emaciation
  - Altered metabolic state
  - Altered circulation
  - Altered sensation
  - Altered pigmentation
  - Skeletal prominence
  - Developmental factors
  - Immunological deficit

Alterations in turgor (change in elasticity)
Excretions/secretions
Psychogenic
Edema

Defining characteristics

Disruption of skin surface
Destruction of skin layers
Invasion of body structures

Skin integrity, impaired, potential

■ **Definition** The state in which an individual's skin is at risk of being adversely altered.

Risk factors

External (environmental)
- Hypothermia or hyperthermia
- Chemical substance
- Mechanical factors
  - Shearing forces
  - Pressure
  - Restraint
- Radiation
- Physical immobilization
- Excretions and secretions
- Humidity

Internal (somatic)
- Medication
- Alterations in nutritional state (obesity, emaciation)
- Altered metabolic state
- Altered circulation
- Altered sensation
- Altered pigmentation
- Skeletal prominence
- Developmental factors
- Alterations in skin turgor (change in elasticity)
- Psychogenic
- Immunological

Sleep pattern disturbance

- **Definition** Disruption of sleep time causes discomfort or interferes with desired life-style.

Related factors

Sensory alterations
  Internal factors
    Illness
    Psychological stress
  External factors
    Environmental changes
    Social cues

Defining characteristics

Verbal complaints of difficulty in falling asleep
Awakening earlier or later than desired
Interrupted sleep
Verbal complaints of not feeling well rested
Changes in behavior and performance
  Increasing irritability
  Restlessness
  Disorientation
  Lethargy
  Listlessness
Physical signs
  Mild, fleeting nystagmus
  Slight hand tremor
  Ptosis of eyelid
  Expressionless face
Thick speech with mispronunciation and incorrect words
Dark circles under eyes
Frequent yawning
Changes in posture
Not feeling well rested

Social interaction, impaired

- **Definition** The state in which an individual participates in an insufficient or excessive quantity or ineffective quality of social exchange.

Related factors

Knowledge/skill deficit about ways to enhance mutuality
Communication barriers
Self-concept disturbance
Absence of available significant others or peers
Limited physical mobility
Therapeutic isolation
Sociocultural dissonance
Environmental barriers
Altered thought processes

Defining characteristics

Verbalized or observed discomfort in social situations
Verbalized or observed inability to receive or communicate a satisfying sense of belonging, caring, interest, or shared history
Observed use of unsuccessful social interaction behaviors
Dysfunctional interaction with peers, family, and/or others
Family report of change in style or pattern of interaction

Social isolation

■ **Definition** Aloneness experienced by an individual and perceived as imposed by others and as a negative or threatened state.

Related factors

Factors contributing to the absence of satisfying personal relationships, such as the following:
- Delay in accomplishing developmental tasks
- Immature interests
- Alterations in physical appearance
- Alterations in mental status
- Unaccepted social behavior
- Unaccepted social values
- Altered state of wellness
- Inadequate personal resources
- Inability to engage in satisfying personal relationships

Defining characteristics

Objective

Absence of supportive significant other(s)—family, friends, group
Sad, dull affect
Inappropriate or immature interests and activities for developmental age or stage
Uncommunicative, withdrawn; no eye contact
Preoccupation with own thoughts; repetitive, meaningless actions
Projects hostility in voice, behavior
Seeks to be alone or exists in subculture
Evidence of physical and/or mental handicap or altered state of wellness
Shows behavior unaccepted by dominant cultural group

Subjective
Expresses feeling of aloneness imposed by others
Expresses feelings of rejection
Experiences feelings of indifference of others
Expresses values acceptable to subculture, but unable to accept values of dominant culture
Inadequacy in or absence of significant purpose in life
Inability to meet expectations of others
Insecurity in public
Expresses interests inappropriate to developmental age or stage

Spiritual distress (distress of the human spirit)

- **Definition** Disruption in the life principle that pervades a person's entire being and that integrates and transcends one's biological and psychosocial nature.

Related factors
Separation from religious and cultural ties
Challenged belief and value system (e.g., result of moral or ethical implications of therapy or result of intense suffering)

Defining characteristics
Expresses concern with meaning of life and death and/or belief systems

Anger toward God (as defined by the person)
Questions meaning of suffering
Verbalizes inner conflict about beliefs
Verbalizes concern about relationship with deity
Questions meaning of own existence
Unable to choose or chooses not to participate in usual religious practices
Seeks spiritual assistance
Questions moral and ethical implications of therapeutic regimen
Displacement of anger toward religious representatives
Description of nightmares or sleep disturbances
Alteration in behavior or mood evidenced by anger, crying, withdrawal, preoccupation, anxiety, hostility, apathy, etc.
Regards illness as punishment
Does not experience that God is forgiving
Unable to accept self
Engages in self-blame
Denies responsibilities for problems
Description of somatic complaints

Suffocation, potential for

■ **Definition** Accentuated risk of accidental suffocation (inadequate air available for inhalation).

Risk factors

Internal (individual) factors
- Reduced olfactory sensation
- Reduced motor abilities
- Lack of safety education
- Lack of safety precautions
- Cognitive or emotional difficulties
- Disease or injury process

External (environmental) factors
- Pillow placed in infant's crib
- Vehicle warming in closed garage
- Children playing with plastic bags or inserting small objects into their mouths or noses

Discarded or unused refrigerators or freezers without doors removed
Children left unattended in bathtubs or pools
Household gas leaks
Smoking in bed
Use of fuel-burning heaters not vented to outside
Low-strung clothesline
Pacifer hung around infant's head
Eating of large mouthfuls of food
Propped bottle placed in infant's crib

Swallowing, impaired

■ **Definition** The state in which an individual has decreased ability to voluntarily pass fluids and/or solids from the mouth to the stomach.

Related factors

Neuromuscular impairment (e.g., decreased or absent gag reflex, decreased strength or excursion of muscles involved in mastication, perceptual impairment, facial paralysis)
Mechanical obstruction (e.g., edema, tracheotomy tube, tumor)
Fatigue
Limited awareness
Reddened, irritated oropharyngeal cavity

Defining characteristics

Observed evidence of difficulty in swallowing (e.g., stasis of food in oral cavity, cough/choking)
Evidence of aspiration

Thermoregulation, ineffective

■ **Definition** The state in which an individual's temperature fluctuates between hypothermia and hyperthermia.

Related factors

Trauma or illness
Immaturity

Aging
Fluctuating environmental temperature

Defining characteristics

Fluctuations in body temperature above or below normal range

See also defining characteristics of hypothermia and hyperthermia

Thought processes, altered

■ **Definition** The state in which an individual experiences a disruption in cognitive operations and activities.

Related factors

Physiological changes
Psychological conflicts
Loss of memory
Impaired judgment
Sleep deprivation

Defining characteristics

Inaccurate interpretation of environment
- Cognitive dissonance
- Distractibility
- Memory deficit or problems
- Egocentricity
- Hyper/hypovigilance
- Decreased ability to grasp ideas
- Impaired ability to make decisions
- Impaired ability to problem solve
- Impaired ability to reason
- Impaired ability to abstract or conceptualize
- Impaired ability to calculate
- Altered attention span—distractibility
- Obsessions
- Inability to follow commands
- Disorientation to time, place, person, circumstances, and events
- Changes in remote, recent, immediate memory
- Delusions

Ideas of reference
Hallucinations
Confabulation
Inappropriate social behavior
Altered sleep patterns
Inappropriate affect

Other possible defining characteristic

Inappropriate/nonreality-based thinking

Tissue integrity, impaired

See also Oral mucous membrane, altered.

■ **Definition** The state in which an individual experiences damage to mucous membrane or corneal, integumentary, or subcutaneous tissue.

Related factors

Altered circulation
Nutritional deficit/excess
Fluid deficit/excess
Knowledge deficit
Impaired physical mobility
Irritants
Chemical (including body excretions, secretions, medications)
Thermal (temperature extremes)
Mechanical (pressure, shear, friction)
Radiation (including therapeutic radiation)

Defining characteristics

Damaged or destroyed tissue (cornea, mucous membrane, integumentary, or subcutaneous)

Tissue perfusion, altered (specify type) (renal, cerebral, cardiopulmonary, gastrointestinal, peripheral)

■ **Definition** The state in which an individual experiences a decrease in nutrition and oxygenation at the cellular level due to a deficit in capillary blood supply.

Related factors

Interruption of flow, arterial
Interruption of flow, venous
Exchange problems
Hypervolemia
Hypovolemia

Defining characteristics

Skin temperature: cold extremities
Skin color
- Dependent, blue or purple
- Pale on elevation, and color does not return on lowering leg
- Diminished arterial pulsations

Skin quality: shining
Lack of lanugo
Round scars covered with atrophied skin
Gangrene
Slow-growing, dry, thick, brittle nails
Claudication
Blood pressure changes in extremities
Bruits
Slow healing of lesions

Trauma, potential for

■ **Definition** Accentuated risk of accidental tissue injury (e.g., wound, burn, fracture)

Risk factors

Internal (individual) factors
- Weakness
- Poor vision
- Balancing difficulties
- Reduced temperature and/or tactile sensation
- Reduced large—or small—muscle coordination
- Reduced hand-eye coordination
- Lack of safety education
- Lack of safety precautions
- Insufficient finances to purchase safety equipment or effect repairs
- Cognitive or emotional difficulties

- History of previous trauma

External (environmental) factors

- Slippery floors (e.g., wet or highly waxed)
- Snow or ice on stairs, walkways
- Unanchored rugs
- Bathtub without hand grip or antislip equipment
- Use of unsteady ladder or chairs
- Entering unlighted rooms
- Unsturdy or absent stair rails
- Unanchored electric wires
- Litter or liquid spills on floors or stairways
- High beds
- Children playing without gates at top of stairs
- Obstructed passageways
- Unsafe window protection in homes with young children
- Inappropriate call-for-aid mechanisms for bed-resting client
- Pot handles facing toward front of stove
- Bathing in very hot water (e.g., unsupervised bathing of young children)
- Potential igniting of gas leaks
- Delayed lighting of gas burner or oven
- Experimenting with chemicals or gasoline
- Unscreened fires or heaters
- Wearing of plastic aprons or flowing clothing around open flame
- Children playing with matches, candles, cigarettes
- Inadequately stored combustibles or corrosives (e.g., matches, oily rags, lye)
- Highly flammable children's toys or clothing
- Overloaded fuse boxes
- Contact with rapidly moving machinery, industrial belts, or pulleys
- Sliding on coarse bed linen or struggling within bed restraints
- Faulty electrical plugs, frayed wires, or defective appliances
- Contact with acids or alkalis
- Playing with fireworks or gunpowder
- Contact with intense cold
- Overexposure to sun, sun lamps, radiotherapy
- Use of cracked dishware or glasses

Knives stored uncovered
Guns or ammunition stored unlocked
Large icicles hanging from roof
Exposure to dangerous machinery
Children playing with sharp-edged toys
High-crime neighborhood and vulnerable client
Driving a mechanically unsafe vehicle
Driving after partaking of alcoholic beverages or drugs
Driving at excessive speeds
Driving without necessary visual aids
Children riding in front seat of car
Smoking in bed or near oxygen
Overloaded electrical outlets
Grease waste collected on stoves
Use of thin or worn pot holders or mitts
Unrestrained babies riding in car
Nonuse or misuse of seat restraints
Nonuse or misuse of necessary headgear for motorized cyclists or young children carried on adult bicycles
Unsafe road or road-crossing conditions
Play or work near vehicle pathways (e.g., driveways, lanes, railroad tracks)

Unilateral neglect

■ **Definition** The state in which an individual is perceptually unaware of and inattentive to one side of the body.

Related factors

Effects of disturbed perceptual abilities (e.g., hemianopsia)
One-sided blindness
Neurological illness or trauma

Defining characteristics

Consistent inattention to stimuli on affected side
Inadequate self-care
Positioning and/or safety precautions in regard to affected side
Does not look toward affected side
Leaves food on plate on affected side

Urinary elimination, altered patterns

See also Incontinence (functional, reflex, stress, total, urge)

■ **Definition** The state in which an individual experiences a disturbance in urine elimination.

Related factors

Sensory motor impairment
Neuromuscular impairment
Mechanical trauma

Defining characteristics

Dysuria
Frequency
Hesitancy
Incontinence
Nocturia
Retention
Urgency

Urinary retention

■ **Definition** The state in which an individual experiences incomplete emptying of the bladder.

Related factors

High urethral pressure caused by weak detrusor
Inhibition of reflex arc
Strong sphincter
Blockage

Defining characteristics

Bladder distention
Small, frequent voiding or absence of urine output
Sensation of bladder fullness
Dribbling
Residual urine
Dysuria
Overflow incontinence

Violence, potential for: self-directed or directed at others

■ **Definition** The state in which an individual experiences behaviors that can be physically harmful either to the self or others.

Risk factors

Antisocial character
Battered women
Catatonic excitement
Child abuse
Manic excitement
Organic brain syndrome
Panic states
Rage reactions
Suicidal behavior
Temporal lobe epilepsy
Toxic reactions to medication

SECTION TWO

Nursing diagnoses: prototype care plans

ACTIVITY INTOLERANCE

Related factors: Sedentary life-style; ineffective pain management; imbalance between oxygen supply and demand.

Audrey M. McLane, Marilyn Wade, and Linda K. Young

Patient goals	Nursing interventions	Expected outcomes
Develop activity/rest pattern consistent with physiological limitations	Assist patient in identifying factors that decrease/increase activity tolerance Develop individualized activity/exercise program Collaborate with patient to tailor medication taking to demands of job-related activities Teach patient to monitor physiological response to activity (e.g., pulse rate, shortness of breath) Teach patient to eliminate/reduce activities that provoke pain or fatigue Teach patient use of exercise log to record exercise, activities, and responses (e.g., pulse, shortness of breath, anxiety) Refer to physician for evaluation of therapeutic regimen	Exercise log indicates patient maintains activity level at 4 mets. or less Monitors physiological response to activity Modifies activities that produce pain Tolerates job-related activities without pain or fatigue Develops strategies to take medications according to plan Engages in regular exercise consistent with activity prescription (i.e., <4 mets.) Makes appointment with physician for evaluation of activity intolerance

	Provide written specifications for duration, intensity, frequency, and met. level of ADLs and recreational activities	
Recognize influence of emotional responses on exercise tolerance	Teach patient/spouse influence of fear/anxiety as it relates to activity tolerance Teach cognitive coping strategies (e.g., imagery, relaxation, controlled breathing) Encourage spouse to learn coping strategies and/or assist by guiding/coaching practice of controlled breathing	Learns/practices relaxation techniques Patient/spouse creates private, quiet place in home for patient to practice relaxation techniques Spouse understands reason for and use of patient's cognitive coping strategies
Use social support network to maintain desired life-style	Teach spouse to help patient pace activities Collaborate with patient/spouse to establish plan of daily activities consistent with desired life-style and which require <4 mets. Encourage patient/spouse to seek assistance with home maintenance activities from friends/neighbors Determine interest of patient/spouse in sexual counseling	Spouse assists with ADLs to prevent activity level exceeding 4 mets. Friends/neighbors help with home maintenance activities (e.g., lawn mowing, putting up storm windows) Patient/spouse prepares priority list of desired recreational activities

References: 6, 73, 85, 96, 103, 128, and 223.

ACTIVITY INTOLERANCE, POTENTIAL

Risk factors: Fatigue/weakness following myocardial infarction (NYHA* Classification I); does not comply with exercise prescription; >15% overweight; poor communication between patient and spouse.

Audrey M. McLane and Marilyn Wade

Patient goals	Nursing interventions	Expected outcomes
Participate in cardiac rehabilitation program	Encourage/negotiate with patient to participate in cardiac rehabilitation program Provide written specifications for duration, intensity, frequency, and met. level of ADLs and recreational activities Assist patient with clarification of values Assist patient in verbalizing anxiety/fear/concerns about engaging in exercise	Attends informational classes for all postmyocardial infarction patients Verbalizes fears about increasing level of activity Patient/spouse clarifies values with assistance from nurse Makes decision to enroll in postdischarge cardiac rehabilitation program
Integrate exercise prescription into ADLs	Teach patient/spouse use of exercise log to record activities, time, duration, intensity, and physiological responses (e.g., pulse rate, shortness of breath, lightheadedness) Teach self-monitoring of heart rate during exercise Teach patient long-term value of increased activity Teach self-evaluation of response to activity, including actions for specific signs and symptoms	Uses exercise log to record distance walked and symptoms experienced Uses written list of activities with met. levels to guide activities Uses conservation techniques for household tasks to have energy available for desired activities

Gradually reduce body weight	Encourage spouse to accompany patient on walks Negotiate with patient to make decision to lose weight Collaborate with dietitian to provide low-calorie snacks and diet sodas Assist patient/spouse with preparation of shopping list for low-calorie meals Dietary referral for diet instruction and for recommending caloric requirements Monitor weight twice a week	Agrees to dietary consultation to begin weight reduction program Disposes of high-calorie snacks kept at bedside Instructs spouse to dispose of high-calorie snacks in cupboards at home Prepares shopping list for low-calorie foods with spouse Sets realistic weekly weight loss goal
Improve communication between patient and spouse	Encourage patient/spouse to participate in postdischarge myocardial infarction support group Refer for sexual counseling if patient/spouse expresses interest Monitor/meet needs of spouse during hospitalization Provide for periods of privacy to permit intimacy between spouse and patient Provide written information about resumption of sexual activity	Patient/spouse decides to participate in postdischarge support group for patients and spouses Patient requests/plans for 1 hour of private time during spouse's visits Patient/spouse shares concerns with nurse about resumption of sexual activity and raises questions about written information

References: 39, 73, 128, 162, 315, 353, and 481.

*NYHA, New York Heart Association Functional Classification of Heart Disease. Class I—No limitation. Ordinary physical activity does not cause undue fatigue, dyspnea, or palpitation.

ADJUSTMENT, IMPAIRED

Related factors: Disability requiring change in life-style; altered locus of control.

Elizabeth Kelchner Gerety and Gertrude K. McFarland

Patient goals	Nursing interventions	Expected outcomes
Modify life-style so as to experience maximum control and independence within limits imposed by changed health status	Provide opportunity for expression of fears of progression of disability and death Encourage identification of current remaining personal strengths and intact roles Provide information and instruction based on an assessment of learning readiness Provide factual information regarding disability, treatment, and prognosis Teach patient and family to differentiate between denial of the *presence* of change in health status and denial of *possible limitations* Recognize influence of premorbid personality and past coping mechanisms on patient's current adaptation Generate hope by assisting patient with identifying previous coping behaviors and support systems used for past problem solving Collaborate with patient to develop an individually tailored health care regimen	Makes future plans that are congruent with changed health status Seeks help from and cooperates with assistance of competent caregivers Demonstrates self-care practices that are within prescribed treatment regimen Verbalizes recognition that choice of self-care practices can influence outcome of health status change Uses strengths and potentials to engage in maximally independent and constructive life-style

	Collaborate with other staff to assist in determining what will aid in control and management of patient's health status change Facilitate compromise where patient's identified goals differ from goals developed by health providers Assess for possible correlation between perceived beliefs of patient's family and patient's willingness to participate in plan of care Encourage patient to maintain a sense of control by: Making decisions related to specific aspects of care Sharing observations of physical status and progress with caregivers Having accountability for selected aspects of care (such as active ROM, wiping secretions from tracheostomy, irrigating colostomy) Assess for possible correlation between family's willingness to support patient's changed life-style and patient's ability to adapt to disability Facilitate communication of topics, by patient and family, that are not related to disability (such as current events, family activities, hobbies, recreational interests)	

References: 62, 133, 137, 142, and 237.

Continued.

ADJUSTMENT, IMPAIRED—cont'd

Patient goals	Nursing interventions	Expected outcomes
Assumes responsibility for using social resources for assistance in ongoing health management	Consistently convey value of self-directive behavior on patient's part Encourage patient and family to explore resources such as Medicare, Medicaid, crippled children's programs, Social Security, and disability insurance Refer patient and family to support groups and self-help organizations for assistance with ongoing informational needs, advocacy issues, and current developments in treatment and research	Uses available community resources and support networks

AIRWAY CLEARANCE, INEFFECTIVE

Related factors: Ineffective coughing; excessive secretions; intubated trachea.

Mi Ja Kim and Mary V. Hanley

Patient goals	Nursing interventions	Expected outcomes
Remove secretions more effectively	Assist and teach patient to deep breathe Position patient to maximize inspiratory muscle length to maximize ventilation (e.g., high Fowler's or sitting position, depending on patient's comfort and hemodynamic status) Ask patient to take slow, deep breaths and assess volume for adequacy (i.e., from FRC to TLC) and sustain breath for several seconds before expiration Provide patient with cues/devices to motivate independent deep breathing exercises (e.g., visual or tactile feedback) Provide hyperinflations (e.g., ambu or anesthesia bag) if patient is unable or too tired to augment tidal volume two- to threefold	Breath sounds are clear following treatments Patient is able to cough up secretions following deep breaths Patient or significant other is able to perform airway clearance procedures

References: 175, 176, 264, 273, 369, and 406.

Continued.

AIRWAY CLEARANCE, INEFFECTIVE—cont'd

Patient goals	Nursing interventions	Expected outcomes
	Adjust frequency of deep breathing exercises according to patient's physiological and psychological status (e.g., five deep breaths every hour while awake and every 4 hours during night)	
	Assist and teach patient to cough after several deep breaths	
	Help patient to assume a comfortable cough position (e.g., high Fowler's with knees bent and a lightweight pillow over abdomen to augment expiratory pressures and minimize discomfort)	
	Remove expectorated secretions from opening of tracheotomy tube using aseptic technique; use clean technique in home; note volume, viscosity, and color of secretions	
	Teach patient alternate cough techniques (e.g., huff or quad) if patient is having difficulty with above method	
	Avoid deep suctioning; if patient can cough secretions to tracheal tube, suction the tube only	
	Perform chest physical therapy maneuvers to drain remote areas of lung by gravity (add percussion, if not contraindicated)	

- Vibrate area of interest during exhalation; be prepared to collect expectorated secretions of suction as described above
- Initiate cough assists (as above) or provide a fast ambu breath to stimulate cough receptors, quickly release hand pressure on bag, and again be ready to collect secretions

Adjust frequency of therapy according to achievement of outcome criteria, target times, and patient comfort

Perform intratracheal suctioning only when secretions are reachable by catheter and patient cannot effectively cough

- Prepare patient for this uncomfortable and potentially traumatic procedure and explain purpose and sequence of maneuvers
- Use aseptic technique during suctioning; clean technique is appropriate in home
- Preoxygenate with 100% oxygen before suctioning
- If patient is spontaneously breathing and has a dominant hypoxic drive to breathe, adjust FiO_2 accordingly

Continued.

AIRWAY CLEARANCE, INEFFECTIVE—cont'd

Patient goals	Nursing interventions	Expected outcomes
	After preoxygenation and hyperinflations, use a sterile catheter one half diameter of tube and apply intermittent negative pressure for less than 15 seconds per pass; reoxygenate and remain with patient until return to baseline vital signs Use minimal cuff inflation; if patient is spontaneously breathing and can swallow oropharyngeal secretions and oral feedings without aspiration, the cuff can be left deflated to minimize tracheal damage Consult physician for adjunctive therapies and further assessment: mucolytics, bronchodilators, antibiotics, fiberoptic bronchoscopy, diagnostic tests (e.g., sputum for culture, sensitivity and Gram stain, chest x-ray)	

	Teach patient or significant other airway clearance procedure and administration of medical adjunctive therapies, as appropriate	
Maintain local and systemic hydration	Provide systemic hydration, which is calculated from patient's intake, output, and body weight Provide humidified gas at 37° C and 100% saturation via ventilator, T-piece connector attached to wide-bore tubing, or tracheotomy mask Remove condensed vapor from inspiratory line p.r.n and change humidifier, connectors, and tubing every day Protect opening from unfiltered ambient air and avoid introduction of foreign objects and blind instillation fluids (e.g., saline)	Tracheal tube is free of plugs Tracheobronchial secretions are easily suctioned or expectorated

ANXIETY

Related factor: Unmet needs.

Gertrude K. McFarland and Thelma I. Bates

Patient goals	Nursing interventions	Expected outcomes
Experience reduced anxiety level	Monitor level of anxiety: State of alertness Ability to comprehend Problem-solving ability Ability to be redirected Narrowing perceptual field Attention focused or scattered Level of intellectual functioning Ability to manage ADLs Appropriateness of response to situation Maintain calm and safe environment Decrease stimuli Talk to and reassure patient Remove harmful objects Encourage involvement in activities depending on level of anxiety Guide participation in self-care Assist patient in identifying possible sources of stress	Demonstrates decreased level of anxiety as evidenced by: Decreased tension Less apprehension Decreased perspiration Ability to maintain eye contact Decreased insomnia Decreased restlessness Ability to relax Not harmful to self or others Ability to discuss anxiety and own behavior Decreased hand tremors Decreased quivering voice Ability to identify possible stressors Increased involvement in activities Increasing ability to monitor own anxiety

	Help patient to connect behavior with feelings Encourage patient to discuss feelings about anxiety Obtain patient's perception of anxiety experienced Help patient to identify how anxiety is manifested through behavior Explore with patient ways of anticipating anxiety	
Demonstrate effective coping skills	Explore coping mechanisms with patient; help patient to identify those coping mechanisms that were successful in decreasing anxiety Help patient to identify adaptive coping mechanisms within patient's own cultural expectations Review problem-solving process: Organize Prioritize Implement Evaluate Teach relaxation techniques Deep breathing: Instruct patient to take slow, deep breaths (eyes may be opened or closed) Repeat and demonstrate as necessary Progressive relaxation: Talk to patient in a soothing voice	Demonstrates effective coping skills as evidenced by: Ability to problem solve Demonstration of relaxation techniques Ability to meet self-care needs Ability to form interpersonal relationships

References: 96, 252, 262, 275, 358, 418, and 430.

Continued.

ANXIETY—cont'd

Patient goals	Nursing interventions	Expected outcomes
	Tell patient to sit or lie in a comfortable position in a quiet area (Patient should close eyes unless that makes him/her uncomfortable.) At periods throughout exercise ask patient to focus on breathing (slow and deep) To begin exercise, instruct patient to get in a comfortable position and imagine being in a quiet, comfortable place (e.g., on a beach, listening to a gentle rain). Then instruct patient to gently tense (for 5 seconds) (without injury) and then relax each muscle group (10 to 15 seconds)	

Begin with toes and feet and move progressively upward—calf of leg, thigh, buttock, lower back, hands (make fist), lower arm, upper arm, shoulders, neck, and ending with face (grimace). After relaxing face, patient should remain quiet for 15 minutes (or as patient can tolerate), concentrating on peace, quiet, and breathing

Instruct patient to use entire exercise or just for areas of tension

Explore with patient ways of meeting needs without increasing anxiety

Maslow's Hierarchy of Needs (1968):

- Physiological needs
- Safety needs
- Affiliative needs
- Esteem needs
- Self-actualization

ASPIRATION, POTENTIAL FOR

Risk factor: Enternal feeding via gastroenteric/gastrointestinal tubes.

Kathryn Hennessy and Mi Ja Kim

Patient goals	Nursing interventions	Expected outcomes
Experience no aspiration	Confirm tube placement after insertion and at regular intervals at least every 4 hours with continuous feeding and prior to each intermittent feeding Confirm initial tube placement by chest x-ray in collaboration with physician Aspirate stomach contents. If needed, check aspirate for acidic pH to confirm initial tube placement. If tube becomes dislodged after feedings are initiated, check aspirate for presence of glucose (Injection of 10 cc of air prior to aspiration may prevent tube from collapsing during aspiration. Positioning patient on right side helps to pool secretion.) Monitor other potential risk factors, such as decreased level of consciousness and sedated state Be aware that coughing, vomiting, and suctioning may dislodge feeding tube	Afebrile Vital signs within normal limits for patient No gastric distention; normal bowel sounds No respiratory distress No complaints of nausea or vomiting

Tape feeding tube securely and monitor tube markings for possible tube migration every 4 hours and prior to each feeding

Assess for gastric retention every 4 hours by:

- Checking gastric residuals. If residuals are 50% greater than prescribed volume, hold tube feeding and recheck residual in 1 hour; notify physician if this occurs for two consecutive measurements of residuals (tube feedings may need to be discontinued)
- Checking abdominal girths serially. Measure from one anterior iliac crest to the other. An increase of 8-10 cm above baseline should be considered significant, and tube feeding should be stopped and physician notified

Assess gastric mobility at least every 4 hours by:

- Auscultation of bowel sounds
- Percussion of abdomen for air
- Assessing for nausea/vomiting
- Assessing for diarrhea/constipation
- Assessing for gastric distention

If there are no bowel sounds, distention is present, and/or there is no nausea/vomiting, the tube feeding should be held and physician notified

References: 21, 53, 231, 312, 384, and 449.

Continued.

ASPIRATION, POTENTIAL FOR—cont'd

Patient goals	Nursing interventions	Expected outcomes
	Maintain proper patient positioning during tube feeding administration Increase head of bed 30-45 degrees during feeding to minimize amount of feeding in stomach If unable to elevate head of bed, turn patient to right side to facilitate passage of stomach contents through pylorus (consider alternative feeding method) Stop tube feeding 30-60 minutes prior to physical activity and procedures that require lowering of patient's head	

	Monitor patient for signs of aspiration (cyanosis, dyspnea, cough, wheezing, tachycardia, fever, massive atelectasis with pulmonary edema, hypoxemia, temperature greater than 38° C for 24 hours) Check vital signs, temperature every 4-8 hours Auscultate breath sounds every 4-8 hours Observe and record color, character of sputum every 8 hours (add blue food coloring to tube feeding) Check pulmonary-tracheal secretions for glucose with reagent strip every 4-8 hours (in high-risk patients). Positive glucose indicates presence of formula in secretions (false-positive may occur with presence of blood in secretions)	

BODY IMAGE DISTURBANCE

Related factor: Difficulty accepting body image postmastectomy.

Gertrude K. McFarland

Patient goals	Nursing interventions	Expected outcomes
Accept body change and incorporate into self-concept so as to maintain positive body image	Assess patient's current perceptions and feelings about mastectomy and resulting body change Assess patient's perception of impact of mastectomy on relationship with spouse Respect patient's need for a period of denial Assist patient in expressing feelings such as anger Encourage talking about mastectomy when patient is able to do so Explore feelings about impact mastectomy has on personal appearance Provide information about cosmetic aids and use of clothing styles Encourage patient to use and participate in support services and groups in the community Offer encouragement Praise constructive problem solving to enhance appearance	Maintains positive body image

References: 288, 292, and 293.

BODY TEMPERATURE, ALTERED, POTENTIAL

Risk factor: Trauma affecting hypothalamus.

Kathryn Czurylo and Mi Ja Kim

Patient goals	Nursing interventions	Expected outcomes
Maintain normothermia	Monitor temperature every 2 hours or use continuous temperature monitoring Monitor other vital signs every 2 hours Administer steriods to decrease edema around area of hypothalamus as ordered Administer antipyretic agents as ordered Adjust environmental temperature to patient's needs if body temperature is altered Adjust patient temperature if body temperature is altered, using cooling mattress and tepid baths or heat mattress and warm blankets as necessary Administer IV fluids at room temperature Continue to monitor and report signs and symptoms of hypo/hyperthermia	No signs or symptoms of hypo/hyperthermia: shivering, pallor, flushing, irritability, seizures Temperature 35.8° to 37.3° C Vital signs within normal limits for patient Serum electrolyte and fluid balance within normal limits

References: 43 and 465.

BOWEL INCONTINENCE

Related factors: Occasional memory loss; inaccessibility of toilet facilities; possible anal sphincter damage.

Audrey M. McLane and Ruth E. McShane

Patient goals	Nursing interventions	Expected outcomes
Establish a regular pattern of bowel elimination	Collaborate with family member and patient to establish area for use of commode on first floor of residence Provide for privacy when using commode Collaborate with family member to develop toileting routine after meals Instruct family member to provide early morning breakfast to stimulate gastrocolic reflex Teach patient pelvic floor exercises and coach practice sessions during each visit Collaborate with family member to arrange for home health aide to provide lunch and assist patient with toileting routine	Accepts use of commode Uses commode after all meals Practices pelvic floor exercises with coaching from nurse and/or family member Episodes of bowel incontinence gradually decrease in frequency

	Teach home health aide how to coach patient with pelvic floor exercises	
Prevent skin breakdown	Teach family member to check rectal area daily for signs of redness Provide patient/family member with written directions for daily skin care Teach family member to monitor all medications including nonprescription medications Provide information about incontinence aids	Perirectal skin is normal in appearance Family member arranges for home health aide to assist with lunch and toileting
Obtain medical evaluation of anal sphincter	Encourage family member to make appointment with physician for evaluation of anal sphincter	Makes and keeps appointment with physician
Increase self-esteem and social functioning	Plan with patient/family member for short trips away from home Encourage use of continence aids Demonstrate sensitivity to patient's feelings about odor and incontinence episodes	Uses protective clothing Absence of fecal odor Participates in social activities at least twice a week

References: 120, 170, 248, 268, 270, 284, and 299.

BREASTFEEDING, INEFFECTIVE

Related factors: Previous history of breastfeeding failure; knowledge deficit; poor infant suck reflex.

Michile C. Gattuso and Mi Ja Kim

Patient goals	Nursing interventions	Expected outcomes
Establish lactation	Initiate teaching to reduce patient's inadequate knowledge about breastfeeding Encourage patient/significant others to verbalize emotional attitudes about breastfeeding Observe for presence of flat or inverted nipples Encourage nipple rolling at least 5 times a day Teach Hoffman technique to be performed before each feeding Use milk cups between feedings Demonstrate techniques to help infant "latch on" correctly Observe infant during feeding for faulty sucking mechanism Demonstrate colostrum expression to entice infant Demonstrate tongue training and suck training techniques Promote appropriate positioning for feeding: side lying, football hold, sitting, or across abdomen	Verbalizes accurate information related to breastfeeding Identifies personal and family support for breastfeeding Able to feed infant with minimal assistance Has adequate milk supply Infant nurses at least every 3 hours for 5-7 minutes on both breasts Infant is satisfied between feedings

Maintain the breastfeeding process	Provide for frequent feedings on demand every 2-3 hours around the clock Do not restrict sucking time Offer both breasts at each feeding; demonstrate burping between breasts Provide suggestions for waking a sleepy baby Plan for reduction of use of supplemental feedings Discourage delaying or skipping of feedings Discuss and observe for signs of adequate let-down reflex Provide for rest periods Discuss breastfeeding diet, such as high-protein, high-calcium diet Discuss implications for using medications while breastfeeding Demonstrate use of assistive devices for infants with problems Provide support and positive reinforcement Identify resources and support groups for breastfeeding Describe how mother can tell if baby is getting enough (e.g., daily weights, level of irritability) Provide anticipatory guidance for developmental changes that affect breastfeeding (i.e., growth spurts, increased crying)	Mother expresses confidence in her ability to handle future situations Mother identifies resources for problems/support

References: 34, 99, 168, 190, 326, 383, and 471.

Continued.

BREASTFEEDING, INEFFECTIVE—cont'd

Patient goals	Nursing interventions	Expected outcomes
	Discuss role of father/significant other while breastfeeding	
	Discuss effects of breastfeeding on sexuality	
Have fewer breast complications	Observe breast for engorgement, warmth, redness of nipple, cracks or fissures in nipple, or anomaly of breast	No evidence of breast/nipple trauma
	Encourage short, frequent nursings	Patient verbalizes minimal breast/nipple discomfort
	Apply warm, moist packs 30 minutes before feeding or encourage patient to take warm showers before feeding	Patient verbalizes/demonstrates breast care techniques
	Massage all around breast, moving from outer margin toward nipple	Patient verbalizes satisfaction with breastfeeding

	Hand express or pump breast to soften areola and make nipple protrude Expose nipples to air dry after each feeding Discourage use of soaps or lotions containing alcohol Apply ointments as prescribed after each feeding Expose nipples to 24-watt bulb for 3-5 minutes after feeding Encourage patient to begin feedings on least sore breast Teach proper technique to break suction of nursing infant Vary position of baby's mouth on breast by changing holding position with each feeding Provide analgesics as prescribed Encourage use of supportive bra 24 hours a day	

BREATHING PATTERN, INEFFECTIVE*

Related factors: Respiratory muscle fatigue; impaired respiratory mechanics.

Mi Ja Kim and Janet L. Larson

Patient goals	Nursing interventions	Expected outcomes
Minimize energy expenditure of respiratory muscles	Teach pursed lip breathing, abdominal stabilization, and controlled coughing techniques; provide optimal care for mechanical assistance (e.g., ventilator) if necessary	Slows respiratory rate, increases tidal volume, and reports decreased dyspnea
Increase inspiratory muscle strength and endurance	Evaluate individual patient's inspiratory muscle for training and, if appropriate, initiate inspiratory muscle training	Increases maximal inspiratory pressure and reports decreased exertional dyspnea
	Monitor oxygen saturation with ear oximeter during training session to verify that patient does not desaturate	
Limit work of breathing	Teach patient to monitor color, consistency, and volume of sputum because respiratory infections increase work of breathing	Reports taking p.r.n. antibiotics when sputum color changes (yellow or green)
	Teach patient name, dosage, method of administration, schedule, and appropriate behavior if side effects occur, and consequences of improper use of medications. Optimal pharmacological therapy will decrease both airway resistance and work of breathing	Reports taking methylxanthines and beta agonists as prescribed
	Induce periodic hyperinflation of lungs with a series of slow deep breaths to increase lung compliance	

	Position patient in upright position as needed (to increase vital capacity)	
Maintain normal respiratory rate, depth, and ratio of inspiratory and expiratory times	Continue to monitor rate and depth of respiration, breath sounds, use of accessory muscles of respiration, and sensations of dyspnea (Clinical manifestations of respiratory muscle fatigue include rapid shallow breathing in the early stages with an increase in $PaCO_2$ and decrease in respiratory rate in the late stages. Accessory muscles of respiration will be employed as the work of breathing increases. Respiratory muscle fatigue magnifies sensations of dyspnea.) Continue to monitor ratio of inspiratory time/total duration of respiration (An increase in the ratio of inspiratory time to total duration of respiration indicates a decrease in respiratory muscle endurance.) Continue to observe for abnormal chest wall motion as indication of respiratory muscle dysfunction (This is manifested by paradoxical motion, which is characterized by expansion of the rib cage and inward motion of the abdomen during inspiration. Asynchronous chest wall motion is characterized by disorganized and uncoordinated respiratory motion.)	Rate, depth, and inspiratory-expiratory ratio of respirations remain within normal limits

References: 31, 44, 81, 145, 239, 334, and 405.

*This care plan is designed for patients with stable chronic obstructive pulmonary disease.

CARDIAC OUTPUT, DECREASED

Related factor: Electrophysiological rhythm disturbance (i.e., bradyarrhythmias [with heart rate ≤ 40/minute] or tachyarrhythmias [with heart rate ≥ 180/minute]).

Margaret J. Stafford and Mi Ja Kim

Patient goals	Nursing interventions	Expected outcomes
Regain normal range of cardiac output	Administer and teach antiarrhythmic agents (e.g., isoproterenol, lidocaine, procainamide, etc.) as appropriate Monitor status of bradyarrhythmias or tachyarrhythmias regularly and consult physician for possible changes in medications, their dosage and frequencies, etc. Watch for possible pulse deficit by regularly checking both apical and radial pulses Select appropriate actions from standing orders and implement with nursing judgment when significant premature ventricular complex (PVCs) such as 2 consecutive PVCs (couplets or pairs), bigeminy, multifocal (6 or more per minute), or R on T pattern develops	Cardiac output level is restored to patient's normal range as manifested by modifications of signs and symptoms Cardiac rhythm and rate are stable and within normal range

	Implement nursing judgment/action on standing orders, such as lidocaine IV bolus and/or drip, 2 to 3 micro drops per minute. Titrate drug according to patient's response; reassure patient, check blood pressure, notify physician, and alter interventions accordingly When ventricular tachycardia develops, consult physician stat; administer lidocaine IV bolus (e.g., 50 to 100 mg) with IV drip using standing orders When symptomatic bradyarrhythmia develops, administer atropine IV per protocol, evaluate patient's response, and consult with physician If complete heart block persists, administer isoproterenol IV drip and prepare for possible pacemaker therapy according to standing orders	
Experience reduced incidence of bradyarrhythmia or tachyarrhythmia	Monitor patient's heart rate and rhythm, blood pressure, respiratory rate, sensorium, and affect during isoproterenol therapy Evaluate patient's other medications for vagolytic effects When lethal arrhythmia such as ventricular fibrillation or cardiac standstill (asystole) develops, defibrillate stat (usually with 300 watts per second) per standing orders and follow routine CPR procedure	Incidence of bradyarrhythmia or tachyarrhythmia is gradually reduced

References: 52, 83, 215, 314, 404, and 432.

Continued.

CARDIAC OUTPUT, DECREASED—cont'd

Patient goals	Nursing interventions	Expected outcomes
Experience less stress, fear, and anxiety	Alleviate or minimize fear/anxiety that may aggravate bradyarrhythmias or tachyarrhythmias Eliminate or modify stressors that would provoke anger and frustrations liable to potentiate bradyarrhythmias or tachyarrhythmias Provide comfort measures and assurance to patients	Verbalizes less fear and anxiety

COMMUNICATION, IMPAIRED VERBAL

Related factors: Psychological barrier; developmental or age-related factors.

Gertrude K. McFarland and Charlotte E. Naschinski

Patient goals	Nursing interventions	Expected outcomes
Attend to appropriate stimuli	Reduce stimuli in order to assist patient in attending to appropriate stimuli, or increase stimuli in order to motivate patient Give clear, simple messages using language patient can understand Teach patient to identify and focus on relevant stimuli Assist in correction of faulty perception	Selects and responds to relevant stimuli Perceives stimuli accurately Demonstrates orientation to time, place, and person
Transmit clear, concise, and understandable messages	Provide means for patient to communicate other than verbally (e.g., paper and pencil) Use facilitative communication techniques when interacting with patient (e.g., reflection) Encourage initiation of conversations Encourage expression of feelings Support attempts to improve communication Assist in mastering developmental level or age-related tasks	Selects and organizes words appropriate to receiver and context Uses effective communication techniques Uses appropriate amount of verbiage Expresses feelings appropriately

References: 152, 289, and 290.

Continued.

COMMUNICATION, IMPAIRED VERBAL—cont'd

Patient goals	Nursing interventions	Expected outcomes
	Teach and support use of effective communication techniques	
	Teach and support use of assertive communication	
Use congruent verbal and nonverbal communication	Match verbal and nonverbal communication during nurse-patient interactions	Demonstrates congruent verbal and nonverbal communication
	Validate meaning of nonverbal communication	Shows congruent nonverbal behaviors
	Point out discrepancies in verbal and nonverbal communication	Balances use of verbal and nonverbal communication
	Point out discrepancies in nonverbal behaviors	
	Point out discrepancies in message sent and context within which it is sent	
	Teach and encourage expression of feelings	
	Increase patient's self-esteem	
	Teach and encourage use of stress reduction techniques	
Send and receive feedback	Encourage interaction with others	Listens actively
	Help patient develop understanding of dynamics of relationships	Examines effects of behavior on others
		Asks for and receives feedback

	Increase patient's awareness of strengths and limitations in communicating with others Help patient examine effects of own behavior Describe, demonstrate, and encourage use of active listening skills Provide feedback to patient Obtain feedback from patient Teach patient to request feedback when communicating with others Help patient to accept and send both positive and negative feedback Support efforts to use feedback	Sends feedback to others Uses feedback in communication process
Experience gratification from communication	Explore feelings that result from communication impairment Provide confirming responses to patient Teach and support use of confirming responses when communicating with others Teach patient evaluation of own and other's communication Demonstrate and support responsibility for communication	Sends and receives confirmation when communicating Reports or shows willingness to assume responsibility for communication Reports satisfaction from communication

CONSTIPATION

Related factors: Daily ingestion of calcium channel blocker (Calan) and diuretic (HCTZ); excessive loss of fluids during strenuous activity 3 times a week; inadequate fluid and fiber in diet.

Audrey M. McLane and Ruth E. McShane

Patient goals	Nursing interventions	Expected outcomes
Obtain relief from effects of constipating medications	Use lubricated gloved finger to break up large masses of hard stool; follow with tap water enema	Obtains immediate relief
	Recommend use of fiber supplement once a day while on constipating medications with increase to twice a day if needed	Takes fiber supplement once a day Reports return to usual pattern of elimination: every 1-2 days
Increase ingestion of fluids and fiber-rich foods	Teach patient to record all intake for 48 hours Analyze eating pattern with patient Recommend diet changes to increase bulk in diet Recommend intake of 8 glasses of water daily with increase to 12+ on exercise days	Eats bran muffin or bread daily Eats one high-fiber vegetable daily Verbalizes increase in fluid intake to 8-10 glasses daily

References: 299, 300, and 301.

CONSTIPATION, COLONIC

Related factors: Weakness; fatigue; restricted mobility (functional level 1)*; preference for nonfibrous foods.

Audrey M. McLane and Ruth E. McShane

Patient goals	Nursing interventions	Expected outcomes
Establish a regular pattern of bowel movements	Suggest trial of Ducolax suppository instead of milk of magnesia Establish toileting routine Teach patient/family importance of immediate response to urge to defecate	Has bowel movement at least every 3 days Stool passes easily Experiences sensation of complete passage of stool Responds immediately to urge to defecate
Increase activity level	Encourage outdoor walking (weather permitting) Increase ambulation distance from 20 ft to 40 ft and then to tolerance level Teach abdominal strengthening exercises Teach active ROM	Walks independently with cane or walker Increases length of walks 10 ft per week Active ROM 3 times a day Exercises abdominal muscles 3 times a day
Modify dietary intake to change ratio of low-/high-fiber foods	Teach patient and caregivers to record all intake for 48 hours Analyze eating pattern with patient and caregivers Review medications for side effect of constipation Recommend diet changes to increase bulk in diet, consistent with financial limitations	Eats bran in some form daily Eats one high-fiber vegetable daily Substitutes whole grain for white bread

References: 25, 56, 299-303, and 364.

*Requires use of equipment or device.

CONSTIPATION, PERCEIVED

Related factors: Cultural/family health beliefs (expect to have daily bowel movement); overuse of laxatives.

Audrey M. McLane and Ruth E. McShane

Patient goals	Nursing interventions	Expected outcomes
Modify cultural family health beliefs with respect to need for daily bowel movement	Confront health beliefs that maintain dysfunctional behaviors	Verbalizes acceptance of bowel movement every 2-3 days
Modify toileting routines	Prescribe lemon juice and hot water every morning for 1-week trial Teach patient use of suppository to stimulate evacuation Teach patient to recognize and attend to stimulus behaviors (i.e., actions/behaviors that stimulate urge to defecate)	Drinks hot liquid before breakfast Reports use of rectal suppository less than once a week
Decrease use of laxatives	Provide instruction about use of bulk and fiber in brown-bag lunches Discuss temporary use of Metamucil to supplement natural fiber in diet Teach patient role of exercise in developing and maintaining acceptable pattern of bowel elimination	Substitutes fresh fruit and vegetable sticks for candy or desserts in lunches Gradually increases walking to 1 mile, 4 times a week

References: 301, 302, 304, and 339.

COPING, DEFENSIVE

Related factors: Stressful event; threat to self-esteem.

Linda O'Brien-Pallas, Margaret I. Fitch, and Gertrude K. McFarland

Patient goals	Nursing interventions	Expected outcomes
Experience defenses that are protected against threat	Support individual's personhood, uniqueness, and right to be involved in decision making Seek to understand individual's perspective of situation and what is stressful or threatening to him/her. Specifically, seek to understand individual patient's sense of self and role expectations of self Gently clarify misconceptions When possible, reduce stressful aspects of event Encourage maintenance of social networks If necessary, confront individual regarding *behaviors* that are harmful to others (e.g., ridicule), but do not try to move patient from defensive stance	Does not suffer further insult to self-esteem

References: 90, 194, 242, and 373.

Continued.

COPING, DEFENSIVE—cont'd

Patient goals	Nursing interventions	Expected outcomes
Move away from use of defensive behaviors	Assist individual in exploring nature and characteristics of the event, its demands, and coping resources required; identify where discrepancies exist between ideal and perceived roles in the situation Help individual to identify desired goals Where possible, reduce stressful aspects of the event and enhance individual's coping abilities through: Setting realistic, concrete goals with individual Identifying specific strategies for achieving goals Setting realistic time frames for reaching goals Reviewing capabilities and learning from past experiences Exploring patterns of thinking (especially negative thoughts) Teaching necessary knowledge and skills Acknowledging accomplishments toward desired goals Maintaining social networks Encouraging expression of fears and concerns	Expresses a realistic appraisal of the event, its demands, and coping resources available Expresses comfort with ideal and perceived roles and competencies to manage situation Verbalizes a sense of personal integrity

COPING, FAMILY: POTENTIAL FOR GROWTH

Related factors: Basic needs sufficiently gratified; adaptive tasks effectively addressed; progress toward self-actualization.

Martha M. Morris and Gertrude K. McFarland

Patient goals	Nursing interventions	Expected outcomes
Actualize growth potential of crisis	Identify changes in family dynamics resulting from crisis Identify changes in individual family members resulting from crisis Discuss with individuals and family goals and experiences that maximize growth potential	Verbalizes changes in family roles/relationships Verbalizes changes in individual attitudes, values, and goals Chooses goals and experiences that foster growth

References: 213, 229, 287, 377, and 433.

Continued.

COPING, FAMILY: POTENTIAL FOR GROWTH—cont'd

Patient goals	Nursing interventions	Expected outcomes
	Provide information as needed to enable individuals/family to develop new goals and methods of achieving them that relate to individuals and total family system Facilitate development of new methods of goal attainment	
Develop broader base of support	Identify patient/family readiness to accept support from additional sources Refer patient/family to appropriate resources Initiate contact if necessary Follow up to assure sustained contact and appropriateness of assistance	Verbalizes interest in contacting others experiencing a similar situation Contacts additional persons/groups when referred Develops additional relationships that provide support during crisis Sustains contact with additional sources

COPING, INEFFECTIVE FAMILY: COMPROMISED

Related factors: Inadequate understanding by a primary person; temporary family disorganization; preoccupation by a significant other who is trying to manage emotional conflicts and personal suffering.

Martha M. Morris and Gertrude K. McFarland

Patient goals	Nursing interventions	Expected outcomes
Develop adequate understanding of situation	Provide adequate and correct information to patient and significant others Discuss "sick role" with patient and significant others Encourage family to have realistic perspective based on accurate information Discuss usual reactions to health challenges such as anxiety, dependency, and depression Provide opportunities for patient to discuss need for support with significant others Monitor areas in which knowledge or understanding is inadequate in relation to patient's health challenge	Verbalizes need for more information or clearer understanding relating to the situation Demonstrates understanding of information given Discusses changes in patient and family as result of health challenge

References: 11, 79, 108, 203, and 287.

Continued.

COPING, INEFFECTIVE FAMILY: COMPROMISED—cont'd

Patient goals	Nursing interventions	Expected outcomes
	Encourage patient and family members to discuss expectations of each other in the situation	
Experience increasing comfort	Maintain as much privacy as possible Provide alternative to patient's room for family discussion Provide information about hospital routines, services, and facilities Encourage family members and significant others to verbalize feelings such as loss, guilt, anger, or relief Use communication techniques that confirm legitimacy of both positive and negative feelings (e.g.,	Displays decreased levels of anxiety as environment is perceived as supportive Verbalizes feelings to health care professionals and other family members

	reflecting feelings ["You seem frightened"], presenting reality ["Many people feel angry during this situation"])	
Cope with changes in family processes	Help family to appraise the situation, including both strengths and weaknesses Help family to identify changes in relationships as a result of patient's health challenge Help family members to recognize role changes needed to maintain family integrity Involve family members in care of patient as much as possible Encourage family members to seek help in adjusting to changes in family process from appropriate sources: friends, clergy, professional health care providers	Identifies changes in family roles and processes as a result of patient's health challenge Recognizes roles to maintain family integrity Assumes new roles as necessary to maintain family integrity Significant others participate in care of patient Seeks help in adjusting to changes in family process from appropriate sources

COPING, INEFFECTIVE FAMILY: DISABLING

Related factors: Dissonant discrepancy of coping styles; highly ambivalent family relationships.

Gertrude K. McFarland and Martha M. Morris

Patient goals	Nursing interventions	Expected outcomes
Achieve accurate understanding of conflict in coping styles	Help significant other(s) and patient to verbalize own perceptions of individual coping styles and areas of conflict Help significant other(s) and patient to identify alternative coping behaviors to minimize conflict in adapting to health challenge Identify areas of conflict in coping styles between individuals and within family unit Monitor individual and family coping styles	Verbalizes perception(s) of coping styles and areas of conflict Identifies alternative coping behaviors that may minimize conflict
Develop alternate coping strategies	Help significant other(s) and patient to focus on present feelings and behaviors Clarify communications between significant other(s) and patient Emphasize positive aspects of present coping strategies	Continues to use positive coping strategies Incorporates alternative coping behaviors in adapting to health challenge

	Assist significant other(s) and patient in practicing alternative coping behaviors through relabeling, role playing, contracting, etc.	
Improve level of complementarity in role relationships	Help patient and significant other(s) to verbalize individual needs and expectations of relationships during present health challenge Help patient and significant other(s) to identify individual strengths and weaknesses in adapting to health challenge Assist patient and significant other(s) in discussing areas where individual strengths, needs, and expectations complement each other in adapting to health challenge Help patient and significant other(s) to identify needs and expectations that are not being met Help patient and significant other(s) to identify strategies to develop complementary relationships in adapting to health challenge Assist patient and significant other(s) in practicing new strategies	Verbalizes individual needs and expectations of relationships Identifies strengths and weaknesses in adapting to health challenge Discusses complementary nature of strengths, needs, and expectations of relationships Identifies areas where needs and expectations are not being met Identifies strategies to aid in developing complementary relationships Incorporates alternative strategies in relationships

References: 12, 79, 153, 287, 321, and 478.

COPING, INEFFECTIVE INDIVIDUAL

Related factor: Inadequate response repertoire.

Gertrude K. McFarland and Evelyn L. Wasli

Patient goals	Nursing interventions	Expected outcomes
Develop social coping skills	Provide appropriate social skills training Specify interpersonal problems patient has had in communicating, especially in expressing feelings Identify collaboratively with patient new behaviors to be learned Engage patient in role playing problem interactions Use a variety of techniques to modify each component of behavior (i.e., facial expression, voice content) Provide positive feedback Designate specific tasks to be completed in real-life settings Seek feedback of results when new behaviors are used in real-life settings Provide attention-focusing skills training Identify area of conversational skill to be developed Begin conversation with patient with a single remark	Demonstrates increased independence Demonstrates increased functional activity Demonstrates decreased social isolation Appropriately expresses ideas, feelings, and needs Uses problem-solving skills Demonstrates assertiveness; is less inhibited Completes everyday tasks involving social skills without development of crises Communicates clearly Demonstrates decreased anxiety Demonstrates ability to perform specific social skills Engages in simple conversational skills

	Praise patient and/or give food or drink to reinforce correct response If patient does not respond correctly then give correct response and repeat remark Reward and reinforce correct response Teach problem-solving skills Have patient role play interpersonal situation Assess patient's receiving skills (i.e., What cues are being attended to? Are various aspects of the situation perceived? Is there an awareness of the relationship aspects of the interaction?) Provide training in specifics to improve receiving skills component of communication process Have patient role play again with purpose of assessing communication processing skills (i.e., What are the options? If X occurs, what factors affect the choice of response? What are the consequences of X?) Provide training in specifics to improve communication processing skills Discuss situation further and assess communication sending skills (i.e., use of tone of voice, facial expressions, body movement, etc.)	Demonstrates decreased use of avoidance, dependency, blaming, bizarre, and aggressive behaviors Reduces use of negativism, social obstreperousness

References: 46, 47, 253, 254, 255, and 278.

Continued.

COPING, INEFFECTIVE INDIVIDUAL—cont'd

Patient goals	Nursing interventions	Expected outcomes
	Provide training in specifics to improve communication sending skills Monitor deficits in social skills as specifically as possible (i.e., lack of assertiveness, poor eye contact, expressionless responses, inappropriate voice tone, inability to converse with others, difficulty with everyday interactions, lack of problem-solving skills, or attention impairments) Evaluate progress in developing social skills to cope with crises at regular intervals	

DECISIONAL CONFLICT (ABOUT SEEKING ANTENATAL GENETIC COUNSELING AND TESTING)

Related factors: Unclear goals and values; uninformed alternatives and consequences; unrealistic expectations.

Annette M. O'Connor and Gertrude K. McFarland

Patient goals	Nursing interventions	Expected outcomes
Select and implement a course of action that is informed, consistent with values, and congruent with behavior	Explore alternatives	Identifies viable alternatives
	Clarify expectations of each alternative	Recognizes consequences of alternatives
	Realign unrealistic or uninformed expectations by providing factual risk information or expert opinion	Expresses realistic probabilities or liklihood of consequences associated with each alternative
	Elicit desirability of each outcome	Identifies positive and negative consequences of alternative actions
	Examine priority of outcomes with patient	Indicates relative importance of each outcome and implicit trade-offs in selection process
	Identify value trade-offs implicit in alternative selection	
	Facilitate alternative selection	Selects course of action consistent with expectations and values
	Assess/teach self-help skills for behavioral implementation of decision	Uses/acquires self-help skills in implementing selected course of action

References: 124, 208, 222, 356, 386, and 417.

DENIAL, INEFFECTIVE

Related factor: Compromised physical status following myocardial infarction.

Linda O'Brien-Pallas, Jane E. Graydon, and Gertrude K. McFarland

Patient goals	Nursing interventions	Expected outcomes
Maintain sense of well-being	Determine patient's degree of denial and effectiveness of same as a coping strategy	Remains defended
	If patient is using full denial, make periodic checks as to patient's stage of denial	
	Support patient's behavior	
	Never directly confront patient's denial	
	Focus on establishing a trust relationship with patient	
	Provide patient with specific information and/or reassurance if he/she should raise any questions or concerns	Expresses some reduction in problems and concerns
	Do not push patient to do this if he/she is not ready (The notion is to work with the patient in terms of his/her particular stage of denial at any point in time.)	

References: 55, 131, 171, 242, 407, 441, and 477.

DIARRHEA

Related factors: Careless food preparation and preservation; infrequent handwashing; family conflict.

Audrey M. McLane and Ruth E. McShane

Patient goals	Nursing interventions	Expected outcomes
Establish a normal pattern of bowel movements	Obtain stool for culture and sensitivity if diarrhea continues Evaluate medication profile for gastrointestinal side effects Teach patient appropriate use of antidiarrheal medications Instruct patient/family members to record color, volume, frequency, and consistency of stools Refer patient for consultation with physician about persistent diarrhea and weight loss	Decrease in number of stools to less than 3 per day Stools are formed Free of abdominal pain

References: 37, 75, 106, 299, 357, 372, and 444.

Continued.

DIARRHEA—cont'd

Patient goals	Nursing interventions	Expected outcomes
Gain weight	Teach patient/spouse how to keep a food diary for 48 hours Evaluate recorded intake for nutritional content Encourage frequent, small feedings (add bulk gradually)	Increases body weight 1 lb per week
Monitor/improve health practices to identify factors contributing to diarrhea	Teach patient to eliminate gas-forming and spicy foods from diet Suggest trial elimination of foods containing lactose Teach/monitor improved handwashing Demonstrate/monitor safe food preparation/preservation Monitor patient/family interactions and environment to identify contributing factors Counsel/teach patient and spouse about healthy conflict resolution strategies	Eliminates irritating foods from diet Eliminates lactose and other suggested food items from diet Makes and keeps medical appointments Practices good handwashing techniques Develops improved practices for food preparation and preservation

DISUSE SYNDROME, POTENTIAL FOR

Risk factors: Immobilization; weakness.

Maureen E. Shekleton and Mi Ja Kim

Patient goals	Nursing interventions	Expected outcomes
Maintain joint movement, muscle size and strength, and bone mineralization	Perform active and passive ROM exercises Dangle at bedside as tolerated Get patient up to chair as tolerated Ambulate as tolerated Anatomic positioning of limbs	Full ROM in joints Muscle size and strength within normal limits
Maintain adequate systemic and local tissue perfusion	Perform bed exercises as tolerated Apply antiembolism stockings Perform positional change in relation to gravity as tolerated: supine → semiupright → upright	BP remains normal and no complaint of dizziness during position changes Peripheral pulses remain intact No dependent edema formation No complaint of weakness/fatigue with activity
Promote feelings of independence and control	Allow opportunity for decision making regarding care Encourage participation in ADLs as tolerated Encourage independence in self-care activities Introduce and encourage use of assistive devices p.r.n.	Patient does not verbalize feelings of powerlessness or loss of control Participates in self-care and ADLs to maximum extent possible

References: 167, 249, and 346.

Continued.

DISUSE SYNDROME, POTENTIAL FOR—cont'd

Patient goals	Nursing interventions	Expected outcomes
		Patient and family/significant others express satisfaction with patient's progress and treatment
Maintain normal skin and tissue integrity	Reposition at last every 1-2 hours Encourage adequate intake of fluids and diet Provide adequate protein in diet Inspect all pressure points at least every 2 hours Provide clean, dry, and wrinkle-free bedding Use assistive pressure relief devices as needed (foam mattress, gel flotation pads, air-fluidized bed, etc.)	Skin remains dry, pink, warm, and intact, especially over bony prominences and pressure points Maintains positive nitrogen balance and tissue hydration
Maintain normal pattern of elimination	Encourage adequate fluid intake Get patient up to bathroom or commode as tolerated—anatomic position to facilitate voiding/defecating	Urine output within normal limits Urine remains clear, light yellow without sediment Urine specific gravity is 1.010-1.025

	Provide adequate roughage in diet as tolerated Provide acid-ash diet Give stool softener/laxative as indicated Provide privacy during acts of voiding/defecation	Bowel movement per regular pattern Stool soft and formed Absence of discomfort when urinating or defecating
Maintain apropriate and adequate sensory stimuli	Provide access to radio, TV, and reading materials Encourage visits from others	Remains oriented to time, person, and place
Maintain effective breathing	Perform deep breathing and coughing exercises every hour Encourage adequate fluid intake Monitor breath sounds	Expectorates secretions Breath sounds clear Tidal volume, NIF, and vital capacity within normal limits Chest excursion is complete and equal bilaterally

DIVERSIONAL ACTIVITY DEFICIT

Related factors: Limited environmental diversional activity; long-term hospitalization.

Gertrude K. McFarland

Patient goals	Nursing interventions	Expected outcomes
Identify strengths and limitations in engaging in diversional activities	Assist patient in describing usual pattern of diversional activities Elicit information about changes desired or required because of altered health status Assist patient in identifying satisfying diversional activities Assist patient in identifying limitations in usual pattern of diversional activities Provide opportunities to continue meaningful diversional activities that are possible within current environment Include patient in making decisions about varying the daily routine	Sets realistic goals for diversional activities Seeks out realistic opportunities for involvement in diversional activities Adapts diversional activities to changing health status

	Plan ample opportunity for visits from friends and family	
Identify strategies for obtaining needed resources	Assist patient in identifying resources needed, space requirements, energy expenditures needed, and nonhuman resources needed (e.g., space) Inform patient about options for diversional activities available in setting (e.g., recreational therapy, occupational therapy, music therapy, art therapy) Support, as possible, patient's perceptions of resources needed for satisfying diversional activity needs	Assumes responsibility for choice of diversional activity
Engage in satisfactory diversional activities	Help patient to identify any changes in ability to engage in chosen diversional activities Adapt environment as possible Encourage patient to verbalize about own experience Provide emotional support and encouragement	Expresses satisfaction with diversional activities

References: 370, 387, and 419.

DYSREFLEXIA

Related factors: Distended bladder, cutaneous stimuli below T7.*

Catherine Ryan and Mi Ja Kim

Patient goals	Nursing interventions	Expected outcomes
Recover from episode of dysreflexia without residual effects	Elevate head of bed or place patient in sitting position Monitor blood pressure and pulse every 5 minutes during acute episode Examine urinary drainage system for obstruction; eliminate obstruction or remove catheter Do not perform Credé's maneuver Catheterize if on intermittent catheter program Assess for signs and symptoms of UTI Loosen tight clothing or restrictive appliances Apply topical anesthetic around anus and in rectum and check for/manually remove fecal impaction Inspect skin for evidence of pressure sore or rashes	Blood pressure and pulse within normal limits for patient Skin dry and without red splotches above level of lesion Absence of pallor below lesion
Recognize symptoms of dysreflexia and seek appropriate treatment	Teach signs and symptoms of dysreflexia Maintain adequate fluid intake Adhere to bowel training program	Experiences no additional episodes of acute dysreflexia

References: 257, 296, and 337.

*Patient has a spinal cord injury (T7 or above) and is at risk for recurrent episodes of dysfunctional autonomic reflex.

FAMILY PROCESSES, ALTERED

Related factor: Situational transition.

Evelyn L. Wasli and Gertrude K. McFarland

Patient goals	Nursing interventions	Expected outcomes
Define problems of individual members in terms meaningful to entire family	Help family describe what is occurring as specifically as possible Identify positive behaviors of family member labeled "bad," "sick," or "rebellious" Help family redefine whole situation in favorable terms (i.e., perceive behavior of each as helpful, as effective in some way, as changeable, and as affirmative)	Demonstrates role congruence Demonstrates clear communication Demonstrates constructive interaction

References: 160, 324, 395, 402, 456, and 468.

Continued.

FAMILY PROCESSES, ALTERED—cont'd

Patient goals	Nursing interventions	Expected outcomes
	Support efforts to clarify the what, who, when, and where among interactions of family	
	Assist members in expressing ideas assertively to resolve problem in responsible manner	
	Assist members in tolerating conflict as problem is redefined and solutions are sought	
Agree on and implement plan to resolve problem	Assist family in exploring options for problem solution	Achieves problem resolution
	Provide information about family dynamics that enhance problem-solving skills of family	Learns new responses to problem
	Assist family in identifying consequences of options for problem resolution proposed	
	Support family members in their efforts to implement problem resolution (e.g., stress related to role change)	

FATIGUE

Related factors: Role strain; increased metabolic demands (lung cancer).*

Audrey M. McLane, Sarah Anne McNabb, and Patricia Saskowski

Patient goals	Nursing interventions	Expected outcomes
Establish a pattern of rest/activity that enables fulfillment of role demands	Help patient to identify excessive demands of caretaker and executive roles	Negotiates reduction of work schedule from 60 to 40 hours per week
	Arrange for additional home health services (e.g., Meals on Wheels for wife's lunch)	
	Formulate with patient options for decreasing work demands (e.g., reduction in work hours, delegation of selected tasks)	
	Help patient to plan a daily schedule that includes pacing leisure activities, rest, and exercise	Walks 2-3 times a week within own and wife's tolerance
		Engages in preferred leisure activities 2-3 times a week
	Monitor level of fatigue using Rhoden Fatigue Scale and Observation Check-list	Verbalizes decreased sense of fatigue
	Counsel wife to enroll in post-stroke home management skills workshop	Spouse enrolls/participates in home management skills workshop

References: 166, 182, 230, 283, 317, 366, and 463.

Continued.

* Patient has lung cancer and is a business executive who has been a caretaker of his wife, who had a stroke.

FATIGUE—cont'd

Patient goals	Nursing interventions	Expected outcomes
	Monitor sleep pattern Teach patient to eliminate/reduce physical activities 1 hour before bedtime	Sleeps a minimum of 6 consecutive hours Feels refreshed on arising
Improve nutritional status	Teach use of food diary to monitor eating habits Review food diary/food preferences Help patient to identify foods high in protein and complex carbohydrates Provide information on use of high-calorie food supplements Teach patient/spouse shortcuts to meal planning and preparation	Stabilizes body weight Consumes well-balanced high-calorie diet—2400 cal
Restore mental energy	Teach/monitor relaxation techniques agreeable to patient (i.e., progressive muscle relaxation, creative imagery, and music) Negotiate use of meditation or prayer	Uses a relaxation technique at least once a day Verbalizes a feeling of renewed interest in life

FEAR

Related factors: Impending surgery with possible pain, loss of control, disfigurement; knowledge deficit; unfamiliarity.

Gertrude K. McFarland and Victoria L. Mock

Patient goals	Nursing interventions	Expected outcomes
Identify specific aspects of impending surgery that are sources of fear	Using techniques of therapeutic communication, encourage patient to verbalize: Subjective feelings experienced Personal perception of danger Perception of own coping skills/limitations Need for assistance from nursing staff	Verbalizes specific fears relating to surgery, realistic perception of danger, own coping ability, and need for assistance
Acquire knowledge/skills for dealing with specific fears	Deal with distorted perceptions Provide information to reduce distortions Encourage specifics rather than generalizations	
	Initiate teaching to reduce inadequate knowledge For unfamiliar environment, orient patient to unit and staff	Verbalizes and displays comfort with unit environment, procedure, and staff
	Teach rationale and procedure for turning, coughing, deep breathing, and leg exercises; allow time for practice and return demonstration	Comfortably demonstrates coughing, deep breathing, and leg exercises Explains events expected to occur preop and postop

References: 71, 179, 328, 381, and 494.

Continued.

FEAR—cont'd

Patient goals	Nursing interventions	Expected outcomes
	Teach specifics for type of surgery (e.g., bowel prep for GI surgery) Teach what to expect postop: recovery room, wound dressings, drains, IV fluids, early ambulation as related to surgery Identify and teach specifics of the surgical experience that the patient would like to know Avoid surprises: tell patient what to expect, especially sensations that will be experienced For fear of pain, teach about postoperative analgesia For fear of loss of control, teach ways of enhancing control (e.g., include patient in planning care; share test results as appropriate) For fear of disfigurement, consider visit by someone who has successfully experienced and is well adjusted to the surgery (e.g., ostomy)	Verbalizes realistic expectations for postoperative period

Engage in adaptive coping	Use available support system to increase comfort and relaxation Include family and significant others in teaching so that they are supportive and knowledgeable, rather than fearful Encourage comforting measures (e.g., music, religious objects, own pajamas, pillow, security blanket if child prefers) Arrange a visit with clergy, if desired by patient Adopt a positive attitude that patient can cope and have a positive surgical experience Facilitate a good night's sleep preoperatively Plan nursing activities to be completed by bedtime Do not wake unless absolutely necessary	Verbalizes increased psychological comfort and coping skills Verbalizes positive attitude toward outcome of surgery Experiences a restful sleep
Experience reduced fear	Continually monitor level of fear (many surgeons will cancel surgery if patient is especially fearful)	Verbalizes decreased fear Pulse and respiration rates are within normal limits

FLUID VOLUME DEFICIT (I)

Related factor: Failure of regulatory mechanisms—hyperglycemic hyperosmotic nonketotic coma (HHNC).

Kathryn Czurylo and Mi Ja Kim

Patient goals	Nursing interventions	Expected outcomes
Maintain adequate fluid volume and electrolyte balance	Monitor vital signs every 15 minutes until stable Administer insulin per order according to blood glucose levels Maintain IV therapy for replacement of fluid per order Administer replacement K+ therapy for hypokalemia as appropriate Monitor I&O every 2 hours; report urine output of less than 1 ml/kg/2 hours Weigh patient daily	Afebrile; BP and pulse within normal limits for patient Glucose under 300 mg/dl I&O balanced Urine specific gravity within normal limits (1.010 to 1.025) Hct/Hgb within normal limits Electrolytes within normal limits Serum osmolarity within normal limits

	Monitor specific gravity of urine every 2 hours Monitor urine electrolytes and report abnormal values Monitor serum electrolytes (especially Na+ and K+), Hct/Hgb, and serum osmolarity and report abnormal values Monitor for circulatory overload during fluid replacement (neck vein distention, rales, dyspnea, S-3, increase in CVP or PAP, tachycardia) Continue to monitor and report worsening fluid volume deficit/electrolyte imbalance signs and symptoms (dilute urine, increased urine output, hypotension, increased pulse rate, decreased skin turgor, increased body temperature, weakness, thirst)	

References: 188, 228, 250, and 420.

FLUID VOLUME DEFICIT (2)

Related factors: Active loss of body fluid.

Mi Ja Kim and Kathryn Czurylo

Patient goals	Nursing interventions	Expected outcomes
Maintain adequate fluid volume and electrolyte balance	Determine cause of active loss and use nursing actions to prevent further loss Monitor vital signs every 1-2 hours Maintain IV therapy for replacement of fluid using colloids, crystalloids, or blood products per order Push p.o. fluids to 2600 ml/day if appropriate Monitor I&O every 2 hours; report urine output of less than 1 ml/kg/2 hours	BP and pulse within normal limits for patient I&O balanced Urine specific gravity within normal limits (1.010 to 1.025) Skin turgor within normal limits Electrolytes within normal limits No restlessness/confusion

Monitor urine specific gravity every 2 hours
Weigh patient daily
Monitor serum electrolytes
Monitor for circulatory overload during fluid replacement (neck vein distention, rales, dyspnea, S-3, increase in CVP or PAP, tachycardia)
Monitor and report worsening fluid volume deficit and/or electrolyte imbalance signs and symptoms (decreased urine output, concentrated urine, output greater than intake, hypotension, increased pulse rate, increased body temperature, weakness, change in mental status)

References: 199, 338, 363, and 434.

FLUID VOLUME DEFICIT, POTENTIAL

Risk factor: Daily use of diuretics.

Mi Ja Kim and Kathryn Czurylo

Patient goals	Nursing interventions	Expected outcomes
Maintain adequate fluid volume and electrolyte balance	Teach patient/family the following: Daily weights and record keeping Record keeping of blood pressure and I&O Importance of maintaining regular schedule of taking diuretics and potassium supplements and eating potassium-rich foods such as bananas, oranges, and raisins Action and side effects of diuretics as necessary Slow position changes to minimize orthostatic hypotension Importance of good nutrition and fluid intake Need to monitor skin turgor and avoid excessive dryness Need to avoid excessively hot environment	Patient/family verbalizes knowledge of monitoring fluid status Serum electrolytes within normal limits Weight within normal limits for patient No excessive thirst

References: 13, 236, and 480.

FLUID VOLUME EXCESS

Related factor: Fluid retention with impaired myocardial contractility.

Mi Ja Kim and Margaret J. Stafford

Patient goals	Nursing interventions	Expected outcomes
Achieve normal level of fluid volume	Administer diuretics as ordered; teach patient the rationale for this medication Weigh patient daily and consult physician to adjust diuretic dosage as necessary Monitor serum level of electrolytes, particularly K^+. If hypokalemia develops, provide potassium-rich diet with appropriate patient teaching and consult physician for potassium supplement as necessary Restrict fluid intake in presence of dilutional hyponatremia with serum Na^+ below 130 mEq/L and monitor I&O daily Provide reduced sodium diet (range 1.2 to 1.6 g daily, if indicated) and teach relationship between high sodium level and fluid retention Offer herbs/spices as an alternative to sodium chloride	Body weight is within patient's normal range Hemodynamic status is restored to normal/acceptable range without medication Electrolyte level stays within normal range Subjective and objective manifestations are improved or alleviated

References: 84, 152, 201, 202, 314, 393, and 480.

Continued.

FLUID VOLUME EXCESS—cont'd

Patient goals	Nursing interventions	Expected outcomes
	Administer and teach about inotropic agents such as digitalis if necessary and ordered Explain and titrate vasopressor agents (e.g., dopamine, dobutamine) and/or vasodilator agents (e.g., sodium nitroprusside, hydralazine) if ordered. Monitor for toxic side effects of drugs Monitor hemodynamic status by reading CVP, MAP, PAP, and PAWP if available; consult physician if values exceed normal ranges Monitor laboratory results relevant to fluid retention (e.g., increased specific gravity, presence of protein	

	urea and granular casts in urine, increased BUN, increased MCV, and decreased hematocrit)	
Experience less discomfort due to excessive fluid volume	Provide position that will allow fluid shift and help alleviate dyspnea (e.g., semi-Fowler's position) Provide support to edematous areas (e.g., pillow under arms and scrotal support) Passive and active ROM exercises if appropriate Provide high-protein and high-calorie diet if indicated Counsel patients if significant changes in sensorium exist or concerns are expressed regarding body image and self-esteem as a result of excessive fluid retention Provide appropriate skin care if edematous and monitor potential for infection	Patient verbalizes less dyspnea and experiences more comfort

GAS EXCHANGE, IMPAIRED

Related factors: Altered oxygen supply; alveolar hypoventilation.

Mary V. Hanley and Mi Ja Kim

Patient goals	Nursing interventions	Expected outcomes
Maintain adequate oxygen supply	Maintain patient airway while awake and asleep Encourage patient to take deep breaths (see Airway clearance, ineffective) Position patient to facilitate ventilation/perfusion matching ("good side down") Remove secretions by coughing or suctioning (see Airway clearance, ineffective) Consult physician regarding supplementary oxygen during activity and/or sleep. If ordered, select devices that enable patient to perform ADLs and teach patient accordingly Counsel patient who has chronic hypoxemia to obtain supplementary oxygen prescription from physician before air travel or trips to high altitude If hypoxemia persists, consult physician for possible mechanical ventilation	Hypoxemia is resolved or improved with or without oxygen supplement or mechanical ventilation Performs techniques that maximize matching Performs ADLs with or without supplemental oxygen

Maintain minimal oxygen demands	If mechanical ventilation is prescribed, monitor ventilator settings, endotracheal and tracheal tube function, and function of ventilator and breathing circuits. Assess patient's ability to wean daily. Initiate weaning and support oxygenation requirements as described above If mechanical ventilation becomes long-term, assess for home management by self or significant others Provide rest periods Schedule activities that will not compete for oxygen supply to vital body functions (e.g., avoid activity immediately after meals) Alleviate or minimize fear/anxiety that may increase oxygen demands Monitor's patient's oxygen response to self-care. If deterioration exists, provide physical care, including full assistance with turning and transfer, and passive ROM exercises Teach patient and significant others self-care that will minimize oxygen consumption (e.g., self-monitoring and pacing techniques for performance of ADLs) Maintain body temperature at patient's normal level to avoid extremes, particularly shivering	Demonstrates energy conservation techniques during ADLs

References: 49, 111, 156, and 455.

GRIEVING, ANTICIPATORY

Related factor: Perceived potential loss of significant person.

Gertrude K. McFarland and Elizabeth Kelchner Gerety

Patient goals	Nursing interventions	Expected outcomes
Participate in constructive anticipatory grief work	Encourage patient and significant others to describe their perceptions of potential loss Encourage verbalization of fears and concerns Determine current sources of social support, such as family, friends, church; disruptions in current life-style that are related to anticipated loss, such as finances, living arrangements, transportation Identify the stage of grieving process that patient and significant others are experiencing During stage of shock and disbelief: Allow for use of denial and other defense mechanisms Avoid reinforcement of denial Provide opportunity for expression of emotions Provide assurance that it is normal to experience intense, chaotic feelings and reactions	Discusses thoughts and feelings related to anticipated loss Appropriate resources (e.g., friends, clergy, support groups, legal consultants, Social Security representatives) are used by significant others Ability to meet ongoing self-care needs is demonstrated by significant others Maintains constructive interpersonal relationships

Avoid judgmental and defensive responses to criticisms of health care providers

Enlist support from others, such as family, friends, clergy

During stage of developing awareness of potential loss:

Provide significant others with ongoing information of patient's diagnosis, prognosis, progress, and plan of care

Encourage significant others to describe desires and information needs in caring for patient

Facilitate significant other's assistance with patient's physical care

Facilitate flexible visiting hours and include younger children where appropriate

Help patient and significant others to share mutual fears, concerns, plans, and hopes with each other

Help significant others to understand that patient's verbalizations of anger should not be perceived as personal attacks

Encourage significant others to maintain their own self-care needs for rest, sleep, nutrition, leisure activities, and time away from patient

References: 113, 151, 174, and 479.

Continued.

GRIEVING, ANTICIPATORY—cont'd

Patient goals	Nursing interventions	Expected outcomes
	Facilitate patient's and significant other's discussion of "final arrangements" (e.g., funeral services, burial wishes, organ donation, wish for autopsy) Evaluate need for referral to resources such as Social Security representatives, legal consultants, or support groups During period of mourning, prior to patient's death: Promote discussion of what to expect when death occurs Encourage significant others and patient to share their wishes in respect to family members being present with patient at time of death	

	Help significant others to accept that a choice to be absent at time of death does not indicate a lack of love or caring for patient Discuss indicators of impending death as appropriate Provide comforting measures for patient; encourage significant others to assist if they wish Encourage significant others to maintain verbal communication and touch with their loved one, even though patient may not respond Provide as much privacy as possible for significant others to be alone or with patient when death is imminent	

GRIEVING, DYSFUNCTIONAL

Related factor: Loss of physiopsychosocial well-being.

Gertrude K. McFarland and Elizabeth Kelchner Gerety

Patient goals	Nursing interventions	Expected outcomes
Demonstrate absence of delayed emotional reactions	Monitor patient's perception of current adaptation, body image, responses from significant others, social network, past life experiences, and past problem-solving skills Provide opportunity for patient to describe experiences that preceded loss of physiopsychosocial well-being Differentiate between helpful and maladaptive use of denial Observe for responses by health care providers that may be reinforcing maladaptive denial by patient Point out reality in a nonthreatening manner without arguing with patient or significant others Present patient with increasing significant facts Clarify and offer missing factual information	Acknowledges awareness of loss Verbalizes thoughts and feelings related to loss

	Facilitate constructive working through of expression of feelings by: Demonstrating tolerance for expression of negative feelings Supporting verbalizations of ambivalence Facilitating contact with persons who can openly express feelings Helping patient to understand possible reasons for feelings Point out universality of need for normal grieving Encourage description of recovery expectations	
Experience resolution of dysfunctional grieving	Evaluate need for referral to resources such as brief psychotherapy, support or self-help groups, family therapy Promote coordination of health team resources to help patient: Develop new skills Make readjustments in life-style Make new emotional investments Encourage description of current and anticipated problems related to loss	Participates in treatment modalities that are recommended for rehabilitation Develops goals that are congruent with loss and that reflect individual values and choices Identifies alternate plans for meeting goals that were significant prior to loss of well-being

References: 241, 365, 429, and 491.

Continued.

GRIEVING, DYSFUNCTIONAL—cont'd

Patient goals	Nursing interventions	Expected outcomes
	Promote patient's recognition of past and present strengths that can be used for coping with current loss Promote description of possible strategies for coping with loss Consider use of role playing to facilitate patient's awareness of possible alternatives and consequences of decisions Facilitate contact with others who have successfully adapted to a similar loss For inpatients, promote use of weekend and daytime passes (based on individual assessment of patient) Provide guidance about available community resources	

GROWTH AND DEVELOPMENT, ALTERED*

Related factors: Inadequate caretaking; environmental and stimulation deficiencies; effects of physical disability.

Carol Kupperberg, Gertrude K. McFarland, and Candice S. Korb

Patient goals	Nursing interventions	Expected outcomes
Reach maximum potential in mental and physical development	Monitor child's developmental progress at regular intervals and support mother and child with praise for each accomplishment Suggest ways to provide appropriate sensory stimulation based on infant's cues—do not overstimulate Monitor nutritional status Assess mother's/caretaker's feeding technique Provide guidance in dealing with feeding problems related to delay in normal progression of oral feeding development Assist/encourage mother/caretaker to select foods that will provide calories and nutrition Monitor height and weight gain at regular intervals	Physical and emotional needs are met

References: 76, 207, 280, and 345.

Continued.

*This care plan is for an infant with fetal alcohol syndrome experiencing motor and mental impairment.

GROWTH AND DEVELOPMENT, ALTERED—cont'd

Patient goals	Nursing interventions	Expected outcomes
Achieve family adaptation	Provide support and reinforce appropriate parenting activities to respond to infant's restlessness, sleeplessness, agitation, frequent crying, and/or resistance to cuddling or holding Facilitate access to well-child care; monitor compliance Assess home for safety hazards Make appropriate referrals to: AA counselor for help with alcohol problem; social worker for financial or employment problems Early intervention program Physical therapist to maximize motor development Nutritionist Agency providing day care or respite care for special-needs children Collaborate with involved professionals	Appropriate supportive services are obtained and used

HEALTH MAINTENANCE, ALTERED

Related factors: Impaired ability to make deliberate and thoughtful judgments; insufficient material resources.

Nancy Creason, Judy Minton, Kim Astroth, and Mi Ja Kim

Patient goals	Nursing interventions	Expected outcomes
Seek help as needed to maintain health	Help patient to clarify health maintenance need Assist patient in defining what help is needed to maintain health Teach patient about helpful resources available in family, community, etc. Help patient to evaluate potential or actual effectiveness of available resources Support patient in establishing contact with appropriate resources Help patient to clarify what factors are impairing ability to maintain health	Clarifies health maintenance needs Defines type of help needed for health maintenance Describes resources Selects helping resources based on evaluation in relation to needs Contacts resources as appropriate Reports use of help as needed to maintain health
Reestablish ability to maintain health	Help patient to evaluate personal strengths and weaknesses that affect health maintenance ability	Identifies factors affecting present altered health maintenance ability

References: 88, 212, and 360.

Continued.

HEALTH MAINTENANCE, ALTERED—cont'd

Patient goals	Nursing interventions	Expected outcomes
	Support patient in organizing and using strengths for health maintenance	Recognizes personal strengths and weaknesses
	Explore with patient ways weaknesses can be improved	Uses strengths to reestablish health maintenance ability
	Teach patient about community resources supportive of health maintenance practices	Works to improve areas of weaknesses
	Monitor patient's progress in reestablishing health maintenance control	Uses community resources appropriately
Monitor and identify further health maintenance needs	Monitor patient's ability to maintain health continuously	Provides input about health maintenance activities
	Educate patient to recognize altered health state	Reports awareness of altered health state
	Help patient to develop behaviors that support health maintenance	Develops effective behavior to support health maintenance
	Collaborate with patient to determine and develop behaviors needed to maintain health	Participates actively in health maintenance activities

HEALTH-SEEKING BEHAVIORS (STRESS MANAGEMENT AND LEISURE)

Related factor: Desire for quality longevity.

Jane Lancour and Audrey M. McLane

Patient goals	Nursing interventions	Expected outcomes
Experience a trusting relationship	Introduce client to Travis' Wellness Inventory and Crumbaugh and Maholick's Purpose in Life Test Promote client's interest in completing Inventory and Life Test Assist client in interpreting findings Help client to identify factors that threaten personal wellness and action that can be taken Discuss with client the interdependent and interactive relationship of present state of well-being to daily behaviors, thinking, attitudes, and beliefs Facilitate verbalization of desire for change; fears, excitement, priorities, goals, possible action	Identifies present state of wellness and areas in life-style that require attention Identifies realistic goals and plans for enhancing health
Experience enhanced self-awareness	Assist client in identifying present stressors: internal processes and external events Assist client in identifying behavioral responses to stress	Verbalizes present patterns of response to stress and use of coping strategies Consistently engages in one self-training approach

References: 91, 342, 361, and 448.

Continued.

HEALTH-SEEKING BEHAVIORS (STRESS MANAGEMENT AND LEISURE)—cont'd

Patient goals	Nursing interventions	Expected outcomes
	Explore client's use of coping stategies and degree of effectiveness Assist client in assessing quality of dietary intake and physical activity program. Share with client the relationship of nutritional status, exercise, and stress management Examine with client the feasibility of using conscious relaxation as a means of taking positive personal control Elicit client's willingness and interest in expanding self-awareness through self-training programs: self-hypnosis, creative visualization, meditation, sound therapy, etc. Share with client the process of integrating selected/desired programs. Provide client with follow-up resource material	Communicates outcomes of engaging in program(s) of choice and modifies approach as desired

	Emphasize importance of consistency, patience, working within unique capacity in carrying out self-training program	
Engage in an enriched leisure style	Ask client to describe current leisure activities using specific examples Ask client to describe leisure interests in life from childhood to present Expand, if indicated, client's awareness of scope of leisure beyond commercialized activity orientation Help client to verbalize present leisure needs/ preferences Challenge client to identify responses/excuses that serve as constraints on time used for leisure Invite client to list 10 desired experiences that coincide with leisure needs/preferences Help client to gain awareness of *why* these particular leisure experiences are important (e.g. rest, discipline, play, aloneness, distraction, self-growth, movement, fitness, etc.)	Compares past and present leisure style Identifies personal reasons for leisure and potential for related experiences Develops and implements an action plan with a balance of leisure experiences in keeping with personal purposes

Continued.

HEALTH-SEEKING BEHAVIORS (STRESS MANAGEMENT AND LEISURE)—cont'd

Patient goals	Nursing interventions	Expected outcomes
	Facilitate prioritizing desired leisure experiences based on importance of functional purpose Analyze with client the desired leisure experiences for overall balance: alone, with other; active, passive; indoor, outdoor; winter, summer; artistic preferences, entertainment preferences, skill/competition preferences; intellectual pursuits, self-development pursuits Promote client's development of an action plan toward expansion of leisure style and enhancement of health	

HOME MAINTENANCE MANAGEMENT, IMPAIRED

Related factors: Unsafe environmental hazards; inadequate knowledge about home safety and hip precautions (postop total hip); self-care deficits (functional levels 2-3).

Audrey M. McLane, Marilyn Wade, Marie Maguire, and Linda K. Young

Patient goals	Nursing interventions	Expected outcomes
Adapt home environment to promote maximum health/ safety	Collaborate with patient to establish a safe environment Assist patient in negotiating rental/purchase and installation of bathtub rails, tub bench, elevated toilet seat, and grab bars Encourage patient to wear nonskid shoes Instruct patient to keep environment well lighted Encourage placement of cordless telephone in bathroom Provide patient with 24-hour emergency number for health care services	Permanently removes loose scatter rugs Removes excess furniture to clear pathways for walker Consistently uses safety aids in bathroom (tub rails, tub bench, elevated toilet seat, and grab bars) Uses cloth utility bag attached to walker for miscellaneous supplies and cordless telephone Keeps hall and bathroom light on during night
Integrate hip precautions into ADLs	Use written instructions to reinforce learning about hip precautions	Avoids extreme flexion of hip >90 degrees (e.g., avoids bending from hip, avoids using standard toilet seat)

References: 134, 197, 274, 329, 374, and 378.

Continued.

HOME MAINTENANCE MANAGEMENT, IMPAIRED—cont'd

Patient goals	Nursing interventions	Expected outcomes
	Monitor integration of hip precautions into performance of ADLs as independence progressively increases Monitor progress and compliance with treatment plan (weekly)	Avoids adduction of hip (e.g., avoids crossing legs) Avoids internal rotation of hip (e.g., avoids lying on side, sleeps on back with pillow between legs)
Progress toward independence in ADLs	Collaborate with patient to arrange for home health services (i.e., home health aid and registered nurse) Arrange for meals on wheels Arrange rehabilitative services in the home (e.g., physical therapy and occupational therapy) Foster gradual independence in self-care Teach patient to pace activities Encourage progressive increase in activities inside/outside the home (with physician approval)	Manages personal grooming with assistance of home health aide 3 times a week Participates actively in performance of ADLs with less assistance over time Correctly and consistently uses adaptive devices to facilitate ADLs Alternates periods of activity and rest Eats a balanced diet Selects/participates in one outside activity a week

HOPELESSNESS

Related factors: Prolonged activity restriction creating isolation; deteriorating physiological condition; long-term stress.

Charlotte E. Naschinski and Gertrude K. McFarland

Patient goals	Nursing interventions	Expected outcomes
Perform self-care activities according to physical ability	Meet self-care needs, such as nutrition, hydration, elimination, sleep or rest, and hygiene, that patient is unable to meet Seek patient input in decisions about self-care activities (e.g., time of bath) Provide assistance through teaching and support so that patient is able to gradually assume responsibility for care Involve patient in self-care, beginning with one activity and adding others gradually Provide positive feedback for successful attempts at self-care	Maintains adequate self-care

References: 316, 399, and 443.

Continued.

HOPELESSNESS—cont'd

Patient goals	Nursing interventions	Expected outcomes
Reduce isolation from environment	Establish contact and rapport with patient Assist patient in identifying enjoyable diversional activities Provide opportunities for patient to spend time with one other person; gradually increase amount of time and number of persons Discuss with patient options for increasing support networks Encourage visits by significant others	Maintains relationships with others Participates in diversional activities Establishes a support network Reports satisfaction from relationships with others
Express feelings	Provide opportunity for patient to express feelings verbally or nonverbally (e.g., writing or drawing) Facilitate expression of feelings by active listening, open-ended questions, reflection Provide opportunity for physical expression of feelings (e.g., punching bag, exercises), when possible Express empathy while communicating belief that patient can act contrary to the way he/she feels	Identifies feelings Expresses feelings both verbally and nonverbally Reports absence of suicidal ideation

	Offer realistic hope through communicating belief that patient has or can learn skills needed to cope with problems Assist patient in identifying person(s) with whom he/she is comfortable sharing feelings Observe for signs of suicidal intent (e.g., sudden behavior or mood change, conversations about futility of life)	
Increase self-esteem	Monitor patient's abilities and strengths Demonstrate unconditional positive regard for patient Assist patient in identifying those roles that can consistently be carried out successfully Assist patient in developing self-care skills that contribute to mastery of environment Encourage patient to identify and participate in experiences he/she finds satisfying Encourage positive self-statements of patient Provide honest praise about patient's successes/accomplishments	Reports increased feelings of confidence and self-worth Identifies strengths and abilities Maintains good grooming habits and personal hygiene
Control or influence self and environment	Encourage independent behavior Allow patient input into decisions about ADLs and health care	Verbalizes increased ability to control or influence self and environment Identifies realistic goals

Continued.

HOPELESSNESS—cont'd

Patient goals	Nursing interventions	Expected outcomes
	Teach patient how to discriminate between controllable and uncontrollable events Assist patient in determining realistic goals Assist patient in identifying alternative ways to cope Assist patient in identifying consequences of implementing identified alternatives Provide relevant information about illness and treatment Teach stress-reduction techniques (e.g., meditation, guided imagery) Teach patient new coping strategies Assist patient in trying out new coping strategies Demonstrate and teach effective communication techniques (e.g., active listening)	Demonstrates effective coping strategies Uses effective communication techniques Demonstrates effective problem-solving skills Reports finding meaning in life

HYPERTHERMIA

Related factor: Exposure to hot environment.

Kathryn Czurylo and Mi Ja Kim

Patient goals	Nursing interventions	Expected outcomes
Maintain normothermia	Monitor temperature and vital signs every hour Apply internal/external cooling measures as appropriate, such as cool sponge bath or cooling mattress Provide IV fluid therapy per order Provide fluids, 3000 ml/24 hours or as ordered Monitor I&O; report if urinary output is less than 0.5 ml/kg/hour Monitor arterial blood gases, blood and urine lab tests, and report abnormalities Administer antipyretics as ordered Provide temperature-controlled, comfortable environment	Absence of hyperthermia signs and symptoms such as tachycardia, hyperventilation, flushed skin, seizures Temperature between 35.8° and 37.3° C Respiration, pulse, and BP within normal limits for patient

References: 129 and 336.

HYPOTHERMIA

Related factor: Exposure to cold environment.

Kathryn Czurylo and Mi Ja Kim

Patient goals	Nursing interventions	Expected outcomes
Maintain normothermia	Slowly rewarm body by internal/external methods as appropriate Monitor temperature using low-reading thermometer Monitor vital signs every hour—continuous monitoring of ECG; report arrhythmias such as bradyarrhythmia and treat per order Administer room temperature or warmed IV solution per order Monitor arterial blood gases Monitor lab values: serum electrolytes, BUN, creatinine, and glucose; report abnormalities Insert indwelling catheter per order and monitor urine output ever 2 hours; report if less that 0.5 ml/kg/hour Provide temperature-controlled, comfortable environment	Absence of signs and symptoms of hypothermia: shivering, cool skin, pallor Temperature 35.8° to 37.3° C Pulse, respiration, and BP within normal limits for patient Warm skin

References: 72, 276, 476, and 499.

INCONTINENCE, FUNCTIONAL

Related factors: Mobility limitations (functional level 1); recent addition of twice-daily diuretic to medical regimen; no established toileting regimen.

Audrey M. McLane and Ruth E. McShane

Patient goals	Nursing interventions	Expected outcomes
Achieve complete continence	Teach/monitor use of voiding/training every 3 hours Provide positive feedback for small decreases in incontinence episodes	Gradual decrease in episodes of incontinence Keeps a log to record episodes of involuntary loss of urine Responds to positive reinforcement
Establish/adhere to toileting routine	Teach progressive use of Kegel's exercises (see description under Incontinence, stress) Teach/monitor use of voiding record to document voiding attempts	Attempts voiding every 2 hours and gradually increases to every 3 to 4 hours Voids before retiring Uses voiding log to record changes in pattern of urination
Modify environment to facilitate continence	Provide patient with list of resources to rent/purchase commode	Accepts use of commode Designates private area for use of commode

References: 17, 78, 285, 340, 435, 437, and 466.

Continued.

INCONTINENCE, FUNCTIONAL—cont'd

Patient goals	Nursing interventions	Expected outcomes
	Assist patient with selection and creation of private area for commode and supplies on first floor of residence Encourage placement of extra telephone near commode	Keeps walking aids and supplies nearby Uses continence aids to protect skin and clothing Wears clothing easy to manage for toileting Keeps lights on in upstairs hallway and bathroom at night
Establish/adhere to diuretic and fluid intake routine	Develop with patient a schedule for taking diuretics and fluids	Takes afternoon diuretic 4 to 5 hours before bedtime

	Monitor medications for drugs that influence bladder tone and/or amount of urine production Determine consistency of use of potassium supplement or foods high in potassium (low potassium level decreases bladder tone)	Drinks 8 oz of liquid with meals, between meals, and 2 to 3 hours before bedtime
Consult physician for medical evaluation if incontinence persists Reestablish social contacts with friends and family	Monitor progress toward complete continence Determine if/when medical consultation is needed Plan with patient and family for short trips away from residence Demonstrate sensitivity to patient's feelings about incontinence episodes Encourage use of continence aids to protect clothing	Makes and keeps medical appointments Shares voiding/incontinence log with physician Leaves home for 1- to 2-hour periods to visit family/friends Gradually returns to usual social activities

INCONTINENCE, REFLEX

Related factor: Neurological impairment: spinal cord lesion that interferes with conduction of cerebral messages above the level of the reflex arc.

Ruth E. McShane and Audrey M. McLane

Patient goals	Nursing interventions	Expected outcomes
Increase predictable voiding times	Establish plan for bladder training Base plan on patient's background, self-care limitations, acceptance of method, extent of patient's awareness/ability to cooperate, type of bladder problem(s), and subsequent urological complications Establish daily routine for voiding consistent with other desired activities	Patient/significant other accepts/participates in bladder training Patient/significant other demonstrates conditioning techniques Rare episodes of incontinence
Maintain skin integrity	Provide written plan to keep skin clean and dry Monitor skin for signs of redness, abrasions, etc. Instruct in use of protective clothing Teach use of external catheter at night Provide information about easy-to-remove clothing	Skin remains intact Uses protective clothing Obtains/uses easy-to-remove clothing
Preserve renal function	Establish cues/reminders to void Monitor color, amount and odor of urine	Urinalysis confirms absence of infection Residual urine <50 ml

	Monitor amount of residual urine Notify physician of signs and symptoms of infection Teach use of fluid intake/voiding record Monitor pattern of fluid intake and fluid preferences Establish written plan for fluid intake (e.g., 200 ml/2 hours)	
Maintain dignity and sense of self-worth	Demonstrate sensitivity to patient's/significant other's feelings Assist in selection/teaching of manual voiding facilitation techniques	Verbalizes satisfaction with bladder regimen Reports concerns about voiding to nurse or physician Absence of offensive odors Uses selected manual voiding techniques
Modify environment to support demands of bladder regimen	Monitor ability to use equipment Provide easy access to toileting facilities Provide materials to keep voiding record Establish plan to gain independence in self-care consistent with limitations Provide consultation/assistance with discharge planning	Collaborates with discharge planning Directs others to provide needed assistance with self-care Sets personal goals for increasing self-care ability Decreases need for assistance with self-care gradually

References: 152, 274, 285, 299, 349, 408, and 466.

INCONTINENCE, STRESS

Related factors: Weak sphincter, pelvic muscles, and structural supports.

Ruth E. McShane and Audrey M. McLane

Patient goals	Nursing interventions	Expected outcomes
Increase pelvic floor muscle tone and sphincter function	Provide patient with simple description of pelvic floor anatomy and function Provide patient with Kegel's pelvic floor exercises Provide patient with Mandelstam's instructions: "Sit or stand. Without tensing the muscles of your legs, buttocks, or abdomen, imagine that you are trying to control passing stool by tightening the ring of muscle around the anus. This will help you identify the back part of the pelvic floor. "When you are passing urine, try to stop the flow, then restart it. Do this every time you empty your bladder. Gradually you will become aware of the front muscles of the pelvic floor.	Performs pelvic floor strengthening exercises 3 times a day for 6 months

	"Working from back to front, tighten the muscles while counting to four slowly." Do this 3 times a day for the next 6 months.	
Reduce incontinence episodes	Teach patient to keep voiding log Monitor number and pattern of incontinence episodes Instruct patient to void by the clock, beginning with 2-hour intervals Instruct patient to lengthen interval between voidings gradually Assist patient in establishing fluid intake pattern to maintain hydration (e.g., 200 ml/2 hours during day)	Keeps voiding record Uses timer to provide cue to void every 2 hours Drinks 6 to 8 glasses of water a day
Increase in self-esteem and social functioning	Provide positive reinforcement for desired behaviors Teach use of continence aids Assist with development of plan for participation in outside activities	Participates in social/recreational activities on a regular basis

References: 65, 115, 117, 270, 285, 299, and 466.

INCONTINENCE, TOTAL

Related factors: Independent contraction of detrussor reflex due to trauma and surgery; possible anatomic fistula; self-care limitations (i.e., functional level 3)*

Ruth E. McShane and Audrey M. McLane

Patient goals	Nursing interventions	Expected outcomes
Achieve a state of dryness satisfactory to patient and caregiver	Establish bladder training program acceptable to patient and caregiver Empty bladder every 2 hours; lengthen interval gradually Teach/monitor use of voiding facilitation techniques (drink water, run water in sink, pour water over perineum, tap area over symphysis pubis, stroke lower abdomen or inner thighs) Demonstrate/monitor catheterization (if indicated)	Patient and significant other/caregiver demonstrate bladder regimen Decrease in episodes of incontinence to <3 times a week
Avoid urological complications	Refer patient for medical evaluation to rule out treatable etiologies Develop/teach method for obtaining a specimen for urinalysis every 3 months and if symptoms of infection develop Monitor color, odor, and amount of urine Establish/implement written plan for fluid intake (e.g., 200 ml/2 hours from 8 AM to 6 PM)	Patient and/or significant other verbalizes measures to prevent urological complications of total incontinence

Maintain skin integrity	Develop/implement written plan for keeping skin clean/dry Monitor skin for signs of redness, abrasions, etc. Demonstrate/monitor use of external catheter at night Demonstrate use of protective clothing Provide information about continence aids Provide information about easy-to-remove clothing	Skin remains intact
Achieve desired level of independence in self-care	Provide written instruction for all elements of bladder training program Teach use of voiding record Establish plan to gain independence in self-care consistent with limitations	Set goals for increase in self-care ability Monitors own fluid intake/voiding patterns and makes adjustments
Maintain patient's/caregivers dignity and feelings of self-worth	Monitor nurse/patient interactions for negative statements about self Teach patient thought stopping and thought substitution techniques Use behavioral approaches acceptable to patient and caregiver Evaluate caregiver's perceived health, sense of well-being, and feelings of burden Discuss with patient/caregiver importance of planning for caregiver's participation in desired recreational/social activities	Patient/caregiver manages bladder elimination with periodic supervision Increase in number of positive self-statements Primary caregiver participates in outside recreational/social activities weekly

References: 77, 152, 285, 299, 349, 408, and 466.

*Requires help from another person and equipment/device.

INCONTINENCE, URGE

Related factor: History of recurrent bladder infections.

Audrey M. McLane and Ruth E. McShane

Patient goals	Nursing interventions	Expected outcomes
Have fewer bladder infections	Obtain midstream voided specimen for urinalysis Encourage patient to obtain complete medical evaluation of symptoms	Laboratory report of urinalysis confirms presence of urinary tract infection Physician rules out neurological, muscular, and obstructive diseases (e.g., detrussor motor instability, prostatic hypertrophy)
Modify diet and fluid intake to maintain adequate acid of urine	Teach patient to drink concentrated cranberry juice and/or take superphysiological doses of vitamin C (in very large doses, vitamin C is not metabolized and is excreted in urine as ascorbic acid) Teach patient to drink 8 oz of liquid with meals, between meals, and in early evening	Drinks concentrated cranberry juice daily Takes superphysiological amounts of vitamin C Drinks 8 oz of fluid with meals, between meals, and in early evening
Establish/adhere to toileting routine	Assist patient with development of toileting routine Teach/monitor use of voiding record	Attempts voiding every 2 hours, with gradual increase to every 3 to 4 hours

	Monitor/evaluate change in voiding pattern	Uses Kegel's exercises regularly to strengthen pelvic floor muscles Uses voiding log to record voiding attempts, practice of Kegel's exercises, and episodes of incontinence Voids before retiring Enrolls in biofeedback training program if medication and other measures fail to reestablish continence
Alter pattern of response to urge to void	Teach patient to alter pattern of response to urge to void, including: avoid rushing to toilet; respond to urge to void by pausing to relax abdominal muscles; proceed at normal pace	Avoids rushing to toilet Responds to urge to void by pausing and relaxing abdominal muscles, then proceeding at a normal pace
Reestablish continence	Provide positive feedback for small decreases in episodes of incontinence Teach patient to continue use of superphysiological doses of vitamin C and fluid intake schedule to prevent recurrence of urinary tract infection Instruct patient to take antibiotics as prescribed Teach patient to obtain midstream urine specimen at first sign of return of symptoms	Episodes of involuntary loss of urine decrease Uses measures to prevent recurrence of bladder infections (e.g., adequate fluid intake, superphysiological doses of vitamin C) Absence of urinary tract infection as confirmed by urinalysis

References: 17, 66, 191, 226, 284, 436, and 466.

INFECTION, POTENTIAL FOR

Risk factor: Suppressed immune system.

Kathyrn Czurylo and Mi Ja Kim

Patient goals	Nursing interventions	Expected outcomes
Experience no infection	Monitor temperature every 4 hours; report elevation Auscultate lungs daily; report abnormalities Weigh patient daily Check body fluids for alterations in color, odor, or consistency Teach patient to choose high-calorie, high-vitamin foods Follow steps for prevention of impaired skin integrity Limit use of aspirin/acetaminophen, which may mask a fever	Negative culture WBC within normal limits for patient Afebrile Other vital signs within normal limits for patient Patient/family verbalizes knowledge of infection prevention

	Encourage daily shower/good oral hygiene Encourage fluids, 2600 ml/day Obtain cultures per order and report abnormalities Monitor results of CBC and report WBC abnormalities Wash hands prior to each contact with patient Use gloves as necessary Discontinue invasive lines as soon as possible Avoid invasive procedures Use strict aseptic technique when performing invasive procedures Prevent patient exposure to infected visitors/staff Use reverse isolation if indicated Teach patient/family above interventions when appropriate	

References: 69, 82, 169, and 173.

INJURY, POTENTIAL FOR

Risk factors: Altered psychological state; emotional lability.

Gertrude K. McFarland

Patient goals	Nursing interventions	Expected outcomes
Not injure self	Foster interpersonal trust Determine presence of personal or environmental risk factors Monitor emotional state—depression, sadness, anger, aggressiveness, suspiciousness Monitor judgment, decision-making ability, and impulse control Determine need for increased supervision Examine environment for possible physical risks and remove hazardous objects from environment as necessary	Remains free from personal injury Demonstrates impulse control and appropriate judgment

	Assist in identifying stressors Monitor stress levels Reduce environmental stimuli (noise level, number of persons present, frustrating situations, etc.) Obtain patient's personal perception of violence Avoid power struggles by permitting choices within reason Determine appropriate interpersonal distance Plan for unpredictable dangerous behaviors of patient to self or to others Determine limits and maintain consistency Administer medications to calm patient if appropriate Determine social network and role of significant others in affecting patient's behavior Monitor patient's response to emotional turmoil in others	Recognizes stressors that may increase risk of injury Seeks protective environment when needed

References: 19, 20, 178, 269, 293, 327, and 442.

Continued.

INJURY, POTENTIAL FOR—cont'd

Patient goals	Nursing interventions	Expected outcomes
	Encourage expression of feelings	Identifies moods that may increase risk of injury
	Teach patient about self-monitoring emotional state in self	
	Teach patient constructive strategies to channel emotions	Engages in constructive activities that channel emotions
	Teach patient stress management techniques	Maintains control of own behavior
	As appropriate, refer to individual or group psychotherapy, support group, counseling, or other resources	Uses previous constructive and recently learned strategies to cope with stress
		Uses appropriate therapies and community resources as needed

KNOWLEDGE DEFICIT (HOME IV THERAPY)

Related factors: New experience; distrust of health care providers; delayed readiness.

Jane Lancour and Audrey M. McLane

Patient goals	Nursing interventions	Expected outcomes
Develop trusting/ helping relationship	Allow sufficient time during each visit for one-to-one interaction Sit quietly with patient and engage in active listening Inform patient regarding time of each scheduled daily visit Instruct patient as to caregiver's availability via phone, between visits, and types of concerns/questions that could be discussed Leave contact person's name for patient to call regarding financial information Document patient's phone calls: time, date, content, and action taken Capitalize on opportunities to compliment and/or praise	Discusses with caregiver fears and concerns about health state, previous experiences with health care delivery, and therapeutic regimen Calls caregiver with questions Seeks assistance/direction for financial insecurities
Develop readiness for learning	Determine competency and comprehension potential for home IV therapy	Identifies past pattern of effective learning

References: 61, 146, 147, 374, and 375.

Continued.

KNOWLEDGE DEFICIT (HOME IV THERAPY)—cont'd

Patient goals	Nursing interventions	Expected outcomes
	Monitor readiness to learn at each visit and determine best methods for teaching/learning Provide specific printed instructions (including pictures) for home IV therapy Establish best approach for teaching: structured, unstructured, or both Use patient teaching flow sheet	Seeks information through active dialogue Uses printed information pieces as reinforcement to learning
Increase knowledge and skill of basic IV therapy	Evaluate home setting for an area to store supplies and for preparing solutions Demonstrate and have patient return demonstration on handwashing technique and aseptic technique Inspect site of IV puncture at each visit Label needle device with date, time, size, and length of catheter Change tubing every 48 hours Complete site care every 48 hours	Demonstrates handwashing procedure and use of aseptic technique Demonstrates correct preparation of IV fluids (i.e., bag labeling, attaching tubing, and clearing the line) Demonstrates correct recording on IV sheet Demonstrates correct discontinuance of IV fluid

	Demonstrate and have patient return demonstration on how to add IV solution Demonstrate and have patient return demonstration on use of infusion pump Demonstrate and have patient return demonstration on discontinuance of IV solution and capping of line Demonstrate disposal of IV equipment in home setting Evaluate patient's disposal of IV equipment Demonstrate method for recording IV therapy Evaluate entries made by patient on IV record	Demonstrates correct method of capping line Disposes of equipment as demonstrated
Offset potential complications	Describe signs and symptoms of infiltration and how it occurs Describe signs and symptoms of phlebitis and basis of its occurrence Instruct in action to be taken if evidence of either infiltration or phlebitis is noted Instruct patient to check IV site and flow rate every 2 hours	Identifies signs and symptoms of infiltration and phlebitis Verbalizes action to take if evidence of infiltration or phlebitis is noted Checks IV site and flow rate every 2 hours during infusion Verbalizes rationale for regulation of flow Verbalizes action to take if uncertain about events

MOBILITY, IMPAIRED PHYSICAL

Related factors: Acute joint pain in right shoulder and left knee; chronic joint pain in left shoulder and right knee (systemic lupus erythematosus); fatigue.

Teresa Fadden, Janet F. Schulte, and Audrey M. McLane

Patient goals	Nursing interventions	Expected outcomes
Protect currently affected (acute) joints while promoting/ maintaining function of joints affected by chronic lupus symptoms	Coach patient through passive ROM before initiating active ROM twice a day Teach patient how to use a walker correctly Assist patient with task analysis of daily activities Provide information about task simplification, assistive devices, and other energy conservation techniques Teach family member safe transfer techniques Provide rests and supports for acutely affected joints	Maintains full ROM in chronically affected joints Rests and supports acutely affected joints

Verbalize satisfaction with communications with health care providers	Promote expression of feelings about meaning/ resolution of symptoms Assist patient in preparing for physician visits Provide information about ways to communicate symptoms clearly	Speaks about illness in a calm manner Verbalizations are not solely focused on symptoms
Improve rest/ activity pattern	Provide egg-crate mattress for patient's bed Suggest back massage at bedtime to promote sleep Counsel patient to limit naps to 2 a day with no sensory stimulation Counsel patient to maintain a regular bedtime	Reports a minimum of 7 hours of uninterrupted sleep for 3 consecutive nights
Improve pain management	Teach patient how to use progressive relaxation as an adjunct to analgesics and warm moist heat p.r.n. and at bedtime	Rates pain as "3" or less on a scale of 10 over a 48-hour period

References: 89, 198, 286, and 500.

NONCOMPLIANCE (THERAPEUTIC REGIMEN)

Related factors: Inadequate knowledge, motivation, and social support; conflict in values; complexity of regimen.

Polly Ryan and Audrey M. McLane

Patient goals	Nursing interventions	Expected outcomes
Demonstrate accurate performance of specific health behavior	Provide detailed specific instruction for specific behavior that needs to be performed (e.g., exercise prescriptions should include frequency, intensity, duration, safety measures, and general guidelines) Provide opportunities to discuss positive and negative feelings toward desired change Accommodate personality characteristics, coping styles, knowledge base, and locus of control when teaching and establishing a therapeutic relationship Correct misconceptions Assist patient with using a structured method of remembering and performing routine aspects of health care regimen (e.g., pill calendars)	Accurately verbalizes knowledge necessary to perform specific health-related behavior Verbalizes, in concrete terms, a plan to carry out desired health-related behavior Verbalizes errors or misconceptions in prior thoughts and/or behavior Compensates for problems with memory, vision, and/or hearing by using alternative materials or resources
Demonstrate behaviors consistent with goals of therapeutic regimen	Provide discussion opportunities or discussion groups that promote patient insight into actual deviance from desired health behaviors and feelings and attitudes toward these behavioral changes	Actively participate in therapy Verbalizes freedom to express feelings and beliefs Sets goals and priorities consistent with therapeutic regimen

	Identify reference groups that may be used to discuss feelings and develop clearer insights into current behaviors Assist patient with clarification of values Instruct in use of reminders (prompts/cues) that remind individual to perform or change a specific behavior Direct the use of self-monitoring of desired behavior, including the following: Identification of target behavior the patient chooses to change Target behavior must be measurable (count, graph, measure) Antecedents and consequences of behavior are identified and strengthened or faded Self-monitoring record is regularly and consistently reviewed Counsel on use of applied analysis of behavior: Self-monitor Identification of alternative behaviors, antecedents, or cues Patient makes specific plans to alter behavior Patient practices new behavior	

References: 102, 183, 391, and 392.

Continued.

NONCOMPLIANCE (THERAPEUTIC REGIMEN)—cont'd

Patient goals	Nursing interventions	Expected outcomes
	Behavior is evaluated by using self-monitor Provide feedback and encourage self-reward	
	Contract with patient for specific, short-term, measurable behavior, rewarding success	
	Collaborative goal-setting interventions may be used for long-term multiple goals	
Use alternative resources and social support	Direct patient to use sources of social support Provide patient with written information identifying resources and community agencies	Identifies help obtained from alternative sources of support
Engage in activities to strengthen and/or maintain coping ability	Provide/direct patient with information/practice of assertiveness training Identify and encourage use of reference groups Teach IMPACT method of problem solving: Interpret, More, Possibilities, Assess, Change, and Test Assist patient in setting personal goals consistent with goals of health care regimen Teach and provide opportunities to practice imagery, relaxation therapy, and thought stopping	Verbalizes behavioral plan to deal with social situations that oppose the therapeutic regimen

NUTRITION, ALTERED: LESS THAN BODY REQUIREMENTS

Related factors: Increased work of breathing; inadequate intake of nutrients in diet; diminished energy reserve.

Audrey M. McLane, Sheila Schilling-Olson, and Colleen M. O'Brien

Patient goals	Nursing interventions	Expected outcomes
Consume a well-balanced, high-calorie diet (2400 cal)	Teach and monitor use of food diary (include family member and patient) Help patient to identify food preferences, including foods high in complex carbohydrates and high in protein Assist family member in planning high-calorie, high-protein meals Encourage family member to avoid overemphasizing diet Teach importance of oral hygiene before meals to enhance taste of food	Establishes a pattern of 4 to 6 small meals per day after rest periods Uses bronchodilators and steroids with food/milk products Gradually increases dietary supplement from 2 to 6 oz twice a day Reports less gastric distress

References: 36, 51, 61, 105, 282, and 421.

Continued.

NUTRITION, ALTERED: LESS THAN BODY REQUIREMENTS—cont'd

Patient goals	Nursing interventions	Expected outcomes
Stabilize weight and then gradually increase to 10% < ideal	Collaborate with patient to establish a scale of weight outcomes from most desirable to least desirable Establish dietary prescription in collaboration with a dietitian Prescribe dietary supplement (take 1 to 2 hours after meals)	Weight stabilizes (acceptable immediate outcome) Achieve weight gain of 1 lb every 3 weeks, increasing to 1 lb every 2 weeks (most desirable outcome)
Establish a pattern of rest/activity that enables participation in desired activities	Teach pacing of ADLs Instruct patient/family member in use of energy conservation techniques Teach appropriate use of oxygen to increase ability to engage in exercise	Rests 1 hour before and after meals Paces ADLs Does active ROM exercises twice a day Practices inspiratory muscle training exercises as scheduled

	Teach/monitor inspiratory muscle-training exercises Teach patient/family member use of exercise log to record distance walked, use of oxygen supplement, and feelings of breathlessness	Uses portable oxygen to gradually increase walking distance by 5 ft increments Establishes a regular bedtime routine Avoids use of stimulating beverages Enrolls in outpatient pulmonary rehabilitation program Engages in outside social activity weekly
Experience reduction of fatigue and anxiety associated with compromised health status	Teach/monitor family member's use of cognitive coping strategies (e.g., relaxation, imagery) Avoid introducing multiple protocols simultaneously Encourage family member to coach patient in use of selected coping strategies Provide information about adjuncts that facilitate learning specific techniques (tapes, books, records, pamphlets)	Uses self-selected cognitive coping strategies before meals and as needed Reports improved sense of well-being

NUTRITION, ALTERED: MORE THAN BODY REQUIREMENTS

Related factors: Age-associated physiological changes; long-established eating habits; no regular pattern of exercise.

Audrey M. McLane, Colleen M. O'Brien, and Marie Maguire

Patient goals	Nursing interventions	Expected outcomes
Achieve gradual weight loss to 5% to 10% over ideal weight	Explore motivation to lose weight; reinforce if necessary Reinforce commitment to lose weight Monitor weight weekly	Loses 1 to 2 lb per week Rewards self for each 5 lb weight loss
Participate in regular exercise	Help patient to develop a pattern of nonfood rewards for each 5 lb weight loss Explain/review use of exercise log Explore option of taking daily walks Offer pamphlets/samples of exercises for the elderly Establish written contract with patient to increase activity level	Engages in regular exercise for 20 minutes 3 times a week Keeps an exercise log
Eat a well-balanced diet	Teach use of food diary for self-monitoring purposes Analyze (with patient) food diary weekly (include food eaten, time of day, surroundings, circumstances, where eating occurs)	Keeps a daily food diary Chooses foods from 4 basic food groups Decreases intake of sweets from daily, to every other day, to twice a week

	Identify low-calorie food preferences Encourage water consumption to 8 glasses a day Make recommendations for dietary changes in collaboration with patient Suggest techniques to change eating behaviors Teach use of cognitive coping strategies (e.g., distraction, thought stopping, etc.) Establish written contract with patient to use techniques to modify eating behaviors	Attends hot meal program 2 to 3 times a week
Wear well-fitting dentures	Assist patient in making dental appointment Explore use of dental aids (e.g., denture adhesives)	Makes/keeps dental appointments
Increase socialization	Explore possible social organizations/outlets with patient Establish a written contract with patient to attend social activities	Joins a social group Participates in one group activity weekly

References: 61, 118, 322, 325, 382, 427, and 483.

NUTRITION, ALTERED: POTENTIAL FOR MORE THAN BODY REQUIREMENTS

Risk factors: Disruption of relationship with significant other; dysfunctional pattern of intake.

Jane Lancour and Audrey M. McLane

Patient goals	Nursing interventions	Expected outcomes
Alter pattern of intake	Develop a method for patient to keep a daily record of intake and cues associated with intake Analyze log weekly to determine relationship of patient's feelings to pattern of intake Identify with patient desired weight Determine desirable weekly loss Develop with patient a diet prescription Evaluate intake patterns for balance in major food groups	Holds present weight for 1 week followed by loss of 1 to 2 lb per week until desired weight is achieved. Limits alcohol intake to one drink, containing no more than 1 oz of alcohol, per week Verbalizes the relationship between experience of loss and pattern of intake

	Alert patient to dangers of using alcohol as a coping strategy	
Increase energy expenditure	Help patient to identify, select, and participate in one or more energy-expending activities 3 times a week Monitor involvement in selected activity(ies)	Schedules/participates in energy-expending diversional activities at least 3 times a week
Engage in relationships/activities that facilitate positive coping	Assist patient in identifying pattern of social relationships using social network tool Help patient to verbalize his/her responses to efforts to increase/strengthen social network	Seeks support and assistance from selected relationships

References: 10, 54, 200, 244, 458, 472, and 483.

ORAL MUCOUS MEMBRANE, ALTERED

Related factor: Trauma associated with chemotherapy.

Rosemarie Suhayda and Mi Ja Kim

Patient goals	Nursing interventions	Expected outcomes
Maintain a comfortable and functional oral cavity	Establish a mouth care regimen before and after meals and at bedtime to prevent infection For severe stomatitis, increase mouth care to every 2 hours and twice at night (NOTE: Omission of oral hygiene for periods of 2 to 6 hours nullifies past benefits of care.) Remove dentures. Brush and cleanse thoroughly. Do not replace in case of severe stomatitis (red, inflamed mucosa, necrotic ulceration, bleeding, pain when eating or talking) Select a powerful spray or small, soft toothbrush for removal of dental debris. To soften toothbrush, soak in hot water before brushing and rinse in hot water during brushing. Rinse well after use and store in cool dry place (NOTE: Toothbrushes may be contraindicated in severe stomatitis, thrombocytopenia, and neutropenia. A finger wrapped in gauze may also help to remove dental debris.)	Mucosa, tongue, and lips are pink, moist, and intact Absence of inflammation, lesions, crusts, or hard debris Absence of infection Verbalizes comfort and feeling of oral cleanliness Swallows and talks without discomfort

Use toothettes or disposable foam swabs to stimulate gums and clean oral cavity (NOTE: Lemon-glycerine swabs cause drying and irritation of the oral mucosa and tooth decalcification. Avoid their use.)

Encourage flossing between teeth twice a day with unwaxed dental floss if platelet levels are above 50,000/mm

Encourage frequent rinsing of mouth with either of the following:

- Sodium bicarbonate solution: 1 pint water, ½ tsp salt, ½ tsp sodium bicarbonate; discard unused mouthwash every 2 days (may have an unpleasant taste and be irritating)
- Warm saline (frequently solution of choice; is not harmful or irritating, but may not be effective in removing hardened crusts or debris)

Plan small, frequent meals; select soft and liquid foods; chilled or room temperature foods are tolerated best. Select mild malts, shakes, and ice cream to supplement nutrition

References: 20, 48, 92-94.

PAIN (ACUTE)

Related factors: Inadequate pain relief from p.r.n. analgesic (2 days after surgery for inoperable cancer); reluctance to take pain medication.

Audrey M. McLane

Patient goals	Nursing interventions	Expected outcomes
Obtain pain relief	Administer narcotic analgesic as appropriate Use a flow sheet to monitor pain (quality, intensity, duration, effects of narcotic(s), and comfort measures) Collaborate with physician to establish a regular schedule for administration of parenteral/oral narcotics Collaborate with physician to provide upward adjustment of dose when substituting oral for parenteral narcotic Teach patient/family to continue scheduled narcotic use at home to maximize pain relief Provide patient/family with verbal/written, accurate information about narcotic analgesics Assist patient/family with downward adjustment of narcotic (if indicated) after discharge/completion of chemotherapy	Verbalizes comfort and pain relief after analgesic is administered Reports 3 to 4 hours of uninterrupted sleep at night Alternates periods of activity/rest

Augment narcotic-induced pain relief through use of selected diversional, relaxation, and other stress reduction strategies	Provide information about various strategies to augment pain relief (relaxation, guided imagery, diversional activities, etc.) Teach/monitor patient use of selected strategies to augment pain relief Test/evaluate use of physical measures, massage, heat, etc., to increase patient comfort Teach patient/family to use daily log of pain and activities to determine what precipitates/relieves pain	Uses music tapes, TV, and radio for diversion Learns/uses progressive muscle relaxation Collaborates with nurse to test/evaluate selected cognitive strategies and physical measures to augment comfort and pain control
Maintain quality of life, hope, and faith	Teach family members ways to assist with ADLs Teach patient/family to plan/pace ADLs Provide positive feedback for small gains in self-care Teach family members to use back massage and other comfort-inducing measures Enable patient/family to make decision about chemotherapy Discuss with patient/family when/how to contact nurse/physician to assist with problem solving after discharge Assist patient with values clarification and realistic goal setting	Increases participation in ADLs gradually by planning and pacing activities Makes fewer statements about fear of drug dependence Plans with family/health team members for discharge, outpatient follow-up, and home care Clarifies values/hopes for the future Sets realistic goals

References: 211, 279, 307, 311, 398, 428, and 453.

Continued.

PAIN (ACUTE)—cont'd

Patient goals	Nursing interventions	Expected outcomes
	Determine if patient desires visits from spiritual advisor Notify pastor/minister of patient's requests for spiritual counseling Provide positive feedback for achievement of daily goals Provide patient/family with information about cancer support groups	Achieves 1 to 2 goals each day Requests/accepts counseling from spiritual advisor
Enhance/maintain loving relationships with family/significant others/friends	Facilitate open communication with family/significant others Help family members deal with their own fears and concerns about the future	Family members/significant others visit regularly Family members demonstrate caring through physical touch and participation in patient care (e.g., back massage)

PAIN, CHRONIC

Related factors: Inadequate knowledge of self-care regimens; overactivity; overweight.

Pamela M. Schroeder and Audrey M. McLane

Patient goals	Nursing interventions	Expected outcomes
Gain knowledge of self-care activities related to pain control	Instruct correct positioning Avoid pillow under knees Strive toward extension of leg when lying in bed Instruct quad set exercises Instruct safe use of heating pad Pace activities Teach difference between activity and exercise Discuss work simplification activities Discuss relationship between weight and joint stress Prioritize daily activities Monitor patient's subjective pain perceptions Consult with physical therapist and occupational therapist for exercise program Discuss relationship of pain and depression Teach purpose, dosage, side effects, and precautions of prescribed medication	Identifies actions that exacerbate pain Identifies actions that reduce pain Incorporates measures that reduce pain Uses health care system appropriately

References: 9, 38, 206, 225, 279, 305, and 398.

Continued.

PAIN, CHRONIC—cont'd

Patient goals	Nursing interventions	Expected outcomes
	Teach early intervention in pain experience so pain does not become uncontrollable Encourage use of several pain interventions Teach/monitor maintenance of a log of daily activities and pain status Monitor ability to modify activities based on pain status Monitor ability to incorporate pain reduction measures Monitor effectiveness of interventions Explain that pain is characteristic of arthritis Review symptoms that require attention of nurse or other health care professionals Monitor feelings of patient and family regarding use of unproven remedies Encourage avoidance of unproven treatments and quack remedies that are expensive, life threatening, and/or used in place of traditional health care systems Instruct in relaxation techniques and stress management	

	Provide information on Arthritis Foundation services and other community resources to assist in identification of unproven remedies	
Reduce weight	Monitor motivation toward weight reduction Monitor present nutritional patterns Monitor body weight Teach weight reduction principles Discuss adherence strategies	Loses 1 to 2 lb per week
Establish realistic goals	Monitor ability to modify or simplify activities, and review goals as pain status indicates Monitor problem-solving abilities Teach decision-making techniques if indicated	Sets priorities
Achieve satisfaction with ability to control pain	Teach pain-reduction strategies Monitor ability to implement pain-reduction strategies Monitor progress toward toward normalization of life-style Monitor perceptions of ability to control pain Acknowledge positive achievements directed toward nonpain-focused activities Monitor ability to set realistic goals and to make progress toward goals Assist patient and family to attain and/or maintain open communication within family unit	Reduces self-focusing on pain

PARENTAL ROLE CONFLICT

Related factor: Home care of child with special technological needs (e.g., ventilator dependence, hyperalimentation, central line care).

Donna M. Dixon, Karen Kavanaugh, Alice M. Tse, and Mi Ja Kim

Patient goals	Nursing interventions	Expected outcomes
Participate in technology-related care	Monitor parents' desired level of participation in care Monitor knowledge base and competency related to equipment and required care Assess level of anxiety related to skill performance Teach equipment operation, maintenance, safety, and necessary backup Teach CPR as necessary Develop plans for ordering supplies and contacting vendors Provide opportunities to master required home care skills while hospitalized Teach factors that increase frequency of complications Review management of acute episodes Evaluate parents' understanding of special care and provide clarification as needed Provide consistent contact with health professionals for information and follow-up	Participates in routine and complex caretaking activity for child Makes independent, safe decisions related to acute episodes of the illness, equipment malfunction, or need for professional assistance Adapts information for development of personal style of performing skills Incorporates child's special care into a routine daily pattern

Express feelings and concerns about role alterations	Monitor parents' perceptions of current situation as they compare with previous parenting behaviors Monitor perceptions of expected role changes Monitor parents' feelings toward child (i.e., guilt, anger, overprotection) Help parents to verbalize any fears, expectations for the future, feelings of isolation, and feelings of overwhelming responsibility Determine extended family and friends' positive and negative reactions to child's situation Assess financial status and concerns and refer to appropriate resources Provide guidance on child's normal growth, development, and nurturance needs Discuss ways to maintain appropriate parent-child relationship Discuss housekeeping, job-related, and other family-related responsibilities Counsel parents to develop strategies for the future to facilitate expression of feelings and concerns Refer to support groups and parents in similar situations as available and as desired by parents	Verbalizes feelings and perceptions of self, role change, fears, and significant others Maintains roles of primary caretaker, educator, protector, and disciplinarian States adequate financial resources are available Experiences minimal health problems related to role stress Maintains desired level of participation with other parents, health professionals, and significant others in developing resources for emotional and physical support Reports decreased level of stress

References: 15, 97, 126, 240, 347, 385, and 474.

Continued.

PARENTAL ROLE CONFLICT—cont'd

Patient goals	Nursing interventions	Expected outcomes
Incorporate technology into family life	Monitor what other family members know about child and assistive technology Help parents to identify specific impact of technology-related care on daily life Help parents to identify necessary life-style changes Help parents to plan and implement necessary physical adaptations in the home Develop plans with parents for acquiring portable equipment for activities outside the home Explore with parents possible involvement of significant others in care	Integrates new patterns of behavior and responsibility into individual and family life Resumes previous patterns of living, such as parents' return to work and/or school Plans and carries out activities outside the home with significant others Identifies support systems for assistance with child's care Maintains marital relationship

	Encourage parents to involve child in age-appropriate self-care and home responsibilities Discuss with parents the importance of arranging personal time for self and as a couple Identify with parents the availability of short-term and long-term social supports for sibling care and respite care Assist parents in meeting demands of other family member's need for information and development Suggest that parents arrange peer contacts and activities for child and siblings Provide anticipatory guidance regarding schooling Encourage parents to make contact with school system to explore options	Spends time alone and with partner to pursue other interests Interacts with peers, schools, and community

PARENTING, ALTERED (ACTUAL/POTENTIAL)

Related factors: Inadequate knowledge; inadequate role identity; unrealistic expectations.

Gertrude K. McFarland and Martha M. Morris

Patient goals	Nursing interventions	Expected outcomes
Provide safe environment for child	Assess degree of risk to child's safety Contact appropriate authorities if child's safety seems jeopardized	Child's safety is maintained
Develop parent-child attachment behaviors	Encourage touching behaviors by parents Encourage play activities between parent and child Encourage age-appropriate caretaking activities by parents	
Acquire adequate knowledge base for effective parenting	Identify knowledge deficits Identify learning readiness and learning capability of parent Provide opportunity for patient to test out new information Create a positive learning environment	Verbalizes desired knowledge about specific aspects of parenting Demonstrates more effective parenting behavior such as maintaining consistent discipline and providing for child's physical, psychological, emotional, and social needs

Acquire realistic expectations of self, spouse, and infant/child within family	Identify present expectations of self, spouse, and infant/child	Verbalizes expectations of self, spouse, and infant/child
	Identify areas of failure to meet self-expectations	Verbalizes areas of failure to meet expectations
	Provide opportunity for patient to express feelings about unmet expectations	Verbalizes own feelings regarding expectations
	Encourage patient to speculate on reasons for expectations being unmet	Acknowledges own responsibility for attempting to meet expectations, as well as realistic limits of self and others
	Help patient to: Develop realistic expectations as result of increased knowledge of normal development and basic needs Develop strategies to increase possibilities of having expectations met (e.g., discussing expectations with partner, identifying steps that must occur in order to meet expectations)	Develops realistic expectations of self, spouse, and infant/child and strategies that increase possibility of having expectations met

References: 196, 232, 309, 464, and 470.

Continued.

PARENTING, ALTERED (ACTUAL/POTENTIAL)—cont'd

Patient goals	Nursing interventions	Expected outcomes
Achieve role identity as parent	Identify major components and priorities within patient's role identity (i.e., child of one's parents; spouse; career identity) Identify patient's perception of specific parenting behaviors Identify source of verbalized "ideal" parenting behavior Observe parent-child interaction for congruency between verbalized "ideal" of parent behavior and actual behavior Provide opportunity for patient to explore role identity through individual counseling and/or group interaction	Acknowledges inadequate incorporation of "parent" as part of role identity Identifies socially expected parenting behavior Verbalizes previous absence of effective role models Verbalizes incongruency between "ideal" parenting behaviors and actual behavior Incorporates concept of "parent" as integral part of role identity

	Provide opportunity for patient to observe/experience effective parenting behaviors Provide opportunity for patient to implement alternative parenting behaviors	Demonstrates learning of additional parenting behavior Experiences satisfaction in parenting that will support incorporation of concept of "parent" into role identity
Experience emotional, social, and physical support	Identify specific areas of needed emotional, social, and/or physical support Identify specific strengths of patient and support systems Encourage patient to express feelings about areas of need Provide information about additional resources available to meet areas of need Act as liason/advocate as needed for patient in obtaining help from appropriate resources	Recognizes realistic limitations of self and support systems Selects appropriate resources to supplement self and support system Learns to activate additional support systems as needed

References: 196, 232, 309, 464, and 470.

PERSONAL IDENTITY DISTURBANCE

Related factors: Maturational crisis; retirement.

Gertrude K. McFarland

Patient goals	Nursing interventions	Expected outcomes

Maintain positive concept of personal identity	Develop trusting relationship with patient
	Assess patient's sense of self
	Encourage patient to verbalize concerns and anxiety
	Clarify misconceptions
	Provide information about retirement process
	Refer to retirement seminars or to retirement counselor
	Assist in problem-solving
	  Identify goals for retirement
	  Assist patient in identifying available resources
	  Assist patient in developing action plan
	Explore with patient behaviors in order to determine whether they are adaptive or maladaptive
	Use role rehearsal to try out new behaviors
	Mobilize social support from significant others
		Positive acceptance of self

References: 118, 288, and 293.

POISONING, POTENTIAL FOR

Risk factors: Large stock of medications stored in bathroom near cleaning supplies; poor lighting in home; reduced vision (cataracts in both eyes).

Audrey M. McLane

Patient goals	Nursing interventions	Expected outcomes
Adapt home environment to reduce risk of accidental poisoning	Collaborate with patient to establish separate storage area for medications	Permanently removes all cleaning supplies from bathroom Discards outdated drugs Selects an appropriate storage area for medications
	Teach patient to keep environment well lighted	Replaces 25- and 60-watt bulbs with larger bulbs where appropriate Keeps hall and bathroom lights on during evening and night

References: 19, 20, and 442.

Continued.

POISONING, POTENTIAL FOR—cont'd

Patient goals	Nursing interventions	Expected outcomes
Establish/adhere to a safe method for taking medications	Help patient to develop a way to accurately identify medications	Uses magnifying glass to check contents of each bottle Sets up medications for 24-hour period in well-lighted area
	Monitor medication taking	Demonstrates agreed-on method to set up medications Counts with nurse amount of medication remaining in containers
Seek medical evaluation of reduced vision	Provide patient with list of medical and financial resources in community Help patient to make appointments Develop plan with patient and family for medical evaluation	Schedules an appointment for visit from social worker Makes/keeps appointment to see ophthalmologist Family members agree to assist with transportation to keep appointments

POST-TRAUMA RESPONSE

Related factors: Temporary loss of mobility (full leg cast [left leg] and right ankle cast); multiple cuts/abrasions/contusions of right arm; overwhelming feelings of guilt/responsibility for auto accident.

Audrey M. McLane

Patient goals	Nursing interventions	Expected outcomes
Develop/use new coping strategies to deal with excessive feelings of guilt	Teach relaxation, thought stopping, thought substitution, and other stress reduction techniques of interest to patient Provide for use of preferred music selections for relaxation and diversion Provide consultation/referral to deal with excessive feelings of guilt Contact family of significant other to obtain information about health status of significant other Arrange for telephone visits/personal visits with significant other Allow for privacy during interactions with significant other Arrange for spiritual counseling (with patient's approval to contact minister/pastor)	Reports 2 to 3 hours of uninterrupted sleep at night Practices thought stopping and thought substitution techniques Practices relaxation with guided imagery Uses music for diversion Schedules regular visits with minister/pastor Maintains relationship with significant other Decreases excessive verbalization of details of accident Requests family members to maintain outside job and social obligations

References: 30, 50, 96, 172, 221, 308, and 423.

Continued.

POST-TRAUMA RESPONSE—cont'd

Patient goals	Nursing interventions	Expected outcomes
	Discuss with family members the need to fulfill outside obligations to avoid adding to patient's feelings of guilt	
Maintain relationships with loved ones and friends	Instruct family about importance of frequent, short visits from family members and close friends Request family members to bring meaningful personal items for patient's use Ask family members to prepare list of telephone numbers of friends/family for easy access Discuss with family an interim interaction approach: answer patient's questions about accident but avoid excessive details, including pictures Provide family members with information about patient's physical status	Accepts assistance of parents and siblings to deal with outside obligations Asks parents to manage insurance/legal aspects of accident Requests visits from spiritual advisor Initiates telephone visits with friends and personal visits with close friends
Maintain structural/ physiological integrity of body systems	Instruct and assist with active ROM in unaffected limbs Assist with passive ROM in affected limbs (within limits imposed by injury) Make small changes in body position every 2 hours	Retains muscle strength in unaffected limbs Retains full ROM in affected limbs Skin remains intact (no redness, abrasions, etc.)

	Monitor/massage pressure-prone areas of skin Monitor warmth, sensation, and movement of fingers and toes in casted extremities Monitor adequate fluid and fiber intake to prevent bladder and bowel elimination problems Provide for adequate intake of fluids and foods high in fiber	Circulation, sensory, and motor functions remain intact in affected limbs Maintains pretrauma pattern of urine and bowel elimination
Use assistive devices to enhance self-care ability	Arrange for physical therapy twice a day to learn crutch walking Guide patient in learning transfer techniques Praise patient for small gains in managing ADLs Monitor for side effects of increased activity (e.g., increased discomfort/pain in affected limbs)	Transfers from bed to wheelchair with assistance of one person Attends physical therapy sessions twice a day to gain muscle strength and learn crutch walking Practices crutch walking with nursing assistance Resumes resonsibility for ADLs gradually within limits of injuries

POWERLESSNESS

Related factors: Health care environment; illness-related regimen; life-style of helplessness.

Gertrude K. McFarland and Mary E. Markert

Patient goals	Nursing interventions	Expected outcomes
Experience an increased sense of control over life situation and own activities	Provide opportunities for patient to express feelings about self and illness Maintain a calm and confident attitude Encourage patient to feel a sense of partnership with health care team Encourage patient's interest and curiosity in differing aspects of care Be sensitive to events that may induce powerlessness (unfamiliar language and environment, uncertainty of health/illness/treatment; unpredictability of therapy outcomes) Provide positive reinforcement for slight improvements in behavior patterns Teach self-monitoring (diary/record keeping) Reinforce patient's right to ask questions	Verbalizes increased sense of power and control

	Acknowledge/accept expression of angry feelings as manifestation of patient's distress Allow for patient's expression of views before providing information/direction Provide opportunities for expression of positive emotions (hope, faith, will to live, sense of purpose) Help patient to be aware of those aspects that are patient controlled and separate from events that are uncontrollable	
Recover reversible impaired functioning and compensate for irreversible loss	Create/modify environment to facilitate patient's active participation in self-care Help patient communicate effectively with other health team members Provide for privacy needs of patient Eliminate unpredictability of events by informing patient of scheduled tests and procedures Engage patient in decision making whenever possible (selection of roommate, ADL/treatment schedule, wearing apparel) Help patient anticipate sensory experiences that accompany procedures	Identifies situations in which powerlessness is felt Engages in problem-solving behaviors Sets goals and tries alternative adaptive behaviors to increase sense of control and power

References: 62, 87, 234, 316, and 443.

Continued.

POWERLESSNESS—cont'd

Patient goals	Nursing interventions	Expected outcomes
	Consider individual locus of control (internal versus external) when planning care Involve patient by having patient determine what aspect of care he/she is ready to learn and when he/she wants to learn it (Patients experiencing high degrees of powerlessness may need very structured approaches, with self-care being taught in small increments to avoid overwhelming the patient.) Provide relevant literature and/or audiovisual material Help patient identify: Strengths and potentials Improvements in condition Mastery of health care Coping mechanisms and power resources Situations in which patient is likely to feel powerless and coping strategies for such situations Specific stressors and planned approaches to diminish anxiety	

Develop expectations for self and future	Alleviate physical discomfort that diminishes energy reserve (inadequate pain management, interrupted sleep, etc.) Decrease surveillance as safety factors and patient's level of functioning permit Support patient's efforts to increase resources (e.g., obtaining data about new technology) Monitor prevalence of negative self-talk and help patient reality-test self-deprecatory comments Involve family members/significant others in plan of care Support patient's involvement with self-help groups when indicated Facilitate continuity of significant roles (return to work, family involvement, leisure activity) As indicated, help patient to find alternative roles, interests, and use of talents	Integrates therapeutic regimen into life-style

RAPE-TRAUMA SYNDROME*

Related factors: Limited follow-up during crisis phase; inadequate support system; failure to connect rape experience with current physical and emotional health.

Audrey M. McLane, Pamela Kohlbry, and Marie Maguire

Patient goals	Nursing interventions	Expected outcomes
Develop spouse/family support	Encourage/facilitate family counseling Provide support opportunities	Spouse expresses warmth and concern
Make realistic decisions about potential health problems	Teach importance of medication regimen Monitor adherence to medication regimen Provide medical referrals Make telephone follow-up calls for missed appointments	Keeps follow-up medical appointments Takes medications in keeping with prescribed regimen
Resume a satisfying life-style	Teach progressive relaxation Collaborate with patient in pacing social activities Monitor/support patient's experiences with legal system	Reports feeling secure Reestablishes intimate relationship with spouse/significant other (including verbal and sexual)

	Provide or refer for sexual counseling Identify/select strategies to protect from future assaults	Participates in selected social activities Maintains contact with legal system
Cope with cognitive and emotional responses to rape	Monitor evolution/resolution of symptoms using Rape Trauma Symptom Rating Scale Encourage verbalization of feelings Teach use of cognitive coping strategies: thought stopping, desensitization, guided imagery, refuting irrational ideas, etc.	Resolves self-blame Verbalizes anger
Return to desired body weight	Determine patient's/family's usual eating pattern Provide information on high-calorie dietary supplement Monitor body weight	Reestablishes normal pattern of eating Body weight increases 1 to 2 lb per week

References: 61, 63, 64, 104, 180, 245, and 330.

*This care plan is for patients experiencing postcrisis intermediate phase (2 weeks to 3 months after rape event).

ROLE PERFORMANCE, ALTERED

Related factors: Absence of significant role models; situational transition.

Gertrude K. McFarland

Patient goals	Nursing interventions	Expected outcomes
Engage in functional role performance	Determine nature of role performance disturbance—role insufficiency, role failure, interpersonal role conflict, role disturbance Determine role of patient in family and among significant others Determine scope and nature of situational transition experienced Determine cultural factors that impact on role expectations and performance Assist patient in identifying strengths and potentials Clarify any misconceptions patient has about ability to engage in constructive role performance Encourage patient to express concerns and feelings about performing current role more functionally Assist patient in identifying consequences of current role performance versus more functional role performance Assist patient in identifying and implementing strategies to deal with situational transition	Specifies behaviors necessary for successful changed role performance Discusses role expectations and changed role performance with significant others Uses constructive strategies to cope with situational transition Expresses satisfaction with newly acquired functional role performance

Clarify appropriate role performance with patient in terms of role behaviors, related values, consequences, and reinforcers received by significant others
Assist patient in identifying constructive role models and encourage interaction with these persons
Teach patient problem-solving skills
Provide necessary and reliable information to facilitate role change. Refer to groups in which patient can identify role models
Encourage patient to emulate behaviors associated with functional role performance
Discuss with and help family and significant others to understand and support role change
Use role playing to teach role behaviors and provide opportunities for role rehearsal
Request feedback about experience
Encourage expression of feelings related to learning and practicing new role behaviors
Encourage expression of negative feelings on experiencing setbacks while rehearsing role
Assist patient in examining situation
Offer praise for successful role rehearsal and avoid criticizing patient

References: 14, 343, and 488.

SELF-CARE DEFICIT (BATHING/HYGIENE, DRESSING/GROOMING, FEEDING, TOILETING)

Related factors: Intolerance to activity; decreased strength and endurance.

Mi Ja Kim and Rosemarie Suhayda

Patient goals	Nursing interventions	Expected outcomes
Perform self-care activities with minimal energy expenditure and risk of injury	Assist patient with self-care activities as necessary Determine energy requriements of self-care activity; identify sources of excessive energy expenditure (length of time and effort required to complete activity; muscle groups involved; ambient environmental conditions) Monitor activity tolerance (NOTE: Heart rate may be a more sensitive indicator of poorly spaced rest periods than other physiological measures.) Position for bathing, eating, grooming, etc. Avoid awkward postures Keep needed objects within easy reach Unless contraindicated, provide commode Assist with those activities patient is unable to perform him/herself Monitor and take precautions to protect from safety hazards	Completes self-care activities without significant change in baseline vital signs or threat to safety; i.e., patient is able to: Bring food from receptacle to mouth Wash body or body parts Put on or take off necessary items of clothing Sit on or rise from toilet or commode Manipulate clothing for toileting Carry out proper toilet hygiene

	In collaboration with patient, develop individualized activity schedule to achieve goal and monitor progress with frequent feedback Include significant other when appropriate Schedule frequent, short pauses or rest periods Rearrange schedule to reduce energy loss Within tolerance levels and unless contraindicated, begin graduated exercise program (NOTE: Exercise may lessen feelings of fatigue.) Provide activities designed to stimulate patient's thought process and involvement Encourage maximum independence Teach and encourage patient to participate in self-care activities Monitor underlying cause of activity intolerance (prolonged alteration in nutrition, rest/sleep, or work/activity pattern; pain; depression; drug response; pathology; etc.) Anticipate activity intolerance in high-risk patient (patient experiencing situational and developmental stressors) Maintain adequate intake of nutrients Provide frequent, small meals/snacks Provide aesthetic ambience	

References: 18, 161, 162, 219, 331, and 362.

SELF-ESTEEM DISTURBANCE

Related factor: Chronic illness.

Gertrude K. McFarland and Elizabeth Kelchner Gerety

Patient goals	Nursing interventions	Expected outcomes
Experience self-worth, self-respect, self-approval, and self-confidence	Help patient to describe effects of illness on daily activities, occupation, and family Convey respect and nonjudgmental acceptance of patient as a person Convey recognition of patient's expertise or knowledge Encourage patient to identify existing strengths and potentials Discourage ruminations on past problems and failures Monitor extent to which patient's family influences patient's perception of self Teach family members to recognize influence of their interactive styles on patient's perceptions of self Encourage decision making in planning and directing own care Help patient to set initial goals that can be achieved within a short period of time Help patient to become involved in actions to meet goals	Achieves goals within family, work, or school environment that reflect awareness of personal talents and limitations Differentiates between relationships that reinforce positive feelings versus relationships that decrease feelings of worth Engages in activities and groups that promote feelings of belonging and acceptance

	Encourage patient to initiate activities in which success can be anticipated Teach patient to create relationships that provide successful social interaction Encourage participation in treatment modalities that emphasize support, acceptance, and belonging Inspire hope by describing situations in which other patients have overcome similar difficulties	
Develop self-care skills necessary for functioning in society	Encourage patient to participate in a treatment modality, such as an ADL group or outpatient rehabilitation program that focuses on learning or relearning how to live independently in community Emphasize the following areas: health and personal hygiene, housing, meal planning and preparation, money management, and leisure time	Demonstrates improved self-care practices, such as: Maintaining good grooming and personal hygiene practices Identifying symptoms and accurately reporting them Responding appropriately to emergency situations Planning and preparing meals Managing money Planning leisure time Obtaining housing appropriate to health situation or limitation

References: 61, 247, 293, 295, and 306.

Continued.

SELF-ESTEEM DISTURBANCE—cont'd

Patient goals	Nursing interventions	Expected outcomes
Increase use of assertive behaviors and communication skills and recognize impact on self-worth	Teach patient assertive communication skills Teach patient to become aware of harmful effects of negative self-talk Teach patient to develop defenses toward attacks on self Assist patient to explore ways to cope successfully with negative criticism	Demonstrates use of appropriate assertive behaviors and communication skills, such as: Receives positive comments affirmatively Conveys self-confidence by looking directly at other person Assumes facial expression congruent with what is being said Uses negotiation skills to achieve personal goals Stands and walks in erect, straight position

SELF-ESTEEM, CHRONIC LOW*

Related factors: Repeated negative and stressful interpersonal relationships.

Joan M. Caley and Gertrude K. McFarland

Patient goals	Nursing interventions	Expected outcomes
Develop more positive self-evaluations	Explore with patient nature of feelings about self and extent of their existence and change over time Help patient describe experiences that make him/her feel worthwhile and good about self Demonstrate empathy Provide accurate feedback and give honest answers to questions Be genuinely interested in and concerned about patient Be nonjudgmental	Does not express self-negating statements Evaluates self as able to deal with events
Engage in constructive interpersonal relationships	Observe pattern of interactions with others Help patient to identify problems in relating to others Suggest that patient keep journal to assist in problem solving and obtaining feedback	Engages in assertive behavior Has ability to engage in meaningful conversation

References: 61, 90, 98, 162, 255, 285, and 421.

Continued.

*Long-standing negative self-evaluation/feelings about self or self-capabilities.

SELF-ESTEEM, CHRONIC LOW—cont'd

Patient goals	Nursing interventions	Expected outcomes
	Teach patient strategies to improve interpersonal relationships, such as: Building self-confidence Developing communication skills Making constructive use of defenses Developing hobbies and interests Developing personal opinions about issues, along with ability to express self assertively to others Assist patient in setting realistic goals to improve interpersonal relationships Role play a variety of ordinary interpersonal encounters Discourage rumination about past failures Encourage involvement in recreational activity groups Encourage participation in recommended support groups	Develops positive interpersonal relationships Evaluates self as able to deal with interpersonal relationships Does not seek excessive reassurance

SELF-ESTEEM, SITUATIONAL LOW

Related factors: Organizational instability; impending job change; interpersonal conflict.

Gertrude K. McFarland and Joan M. Caley

Patient goals	Nursing interventions	Expected outcomes
Regain previous positive self-evaluation	Help patient to identify changes in feelings about self Assist patient in clearly describing previous state of positive self-evaluation Explore with patient current employment organizational environment, such as: Degree of organizational instability Level of interpersonal conflict Impending threat to current job Assist patient in describing current level of on-the-job performance and any impact on other aspects of daily living Help patient to identify previous problem-solving strategies and strengths and potentials	Does not verbalize negative feelings about self Exhibits confidence in handling job situation Uses constructive conflict resolution skills Able to problem solve, set goals, and take action

References: 61, 90, 154, 285, and 421.

Continued.

SELF-ESTEEM, SITUATIONAL LOW—cont'd

Patient goals	Nursing interventions	Expected outcomes
	Help patient to assess realistic options for self in current organization Discuss and explore other alternatives with patient Offer hope that situation can be handled by describing others who have overcome similar job instabilities Engage patient in problem solving Assess realities of situation Examine personal assets and strengths Identify incremental goals Develop action plan to meet goals	

	Suggest that patient keep journal to assist in problem solving and obtaining feedback Review with patient community groups that could help patient with problem solving and decision making about transitions Offer patient reading materials that might assist in problem solving Support patient's decision-making efforts Teach patient awareness of potential harmful effects of negative self-talk Demonstrate empathy Teach conflict resolution skills Teach patient defenses against attacks from others Refer to resources available identifying job openings	

SENSORY/PERCEPTUAL ALTERATIONS (AUDITORY)

Related factors: Altered sensory reception/transmission/integration; psychological stress.

Evelyn L. Wasli and Gertrude K. McFarland

Patient goals	Nursing interventions	Expected outcomes
Increase skill in reality testing	Assist patient in sharing ideas and feelings by asking questions, listening, sharing experiences, and describing events Be available for patient in a variety of daily living situations so that his/her experiences can be explored and questions answered Assist patient in identifying what, who, when, where, and how of auditory hallucinations Engage patient in a variety of work activities and determine which are successful in reducing auditory hallucinations Teach patient not only to use diversional techniques, but also to think about or focus on some aspect of the environment or diversional technique Avoid suggesting that a voice is being heard	Separates imaginary events from real events Oriented to time, place, and person Absence of auditory hallucination Decreased anxiety level Uses diversional activities to lessen hallucinations Explores environment (i.e., asks questions: what, who, when, where, how) Seeks to experience things/events for self

References: 7, 33, 109, 214, 272, and 498.

SEXUAL DYSFUNCTION

Related factors: Misinformation or inadequate knowledge; values conflict.

Gertrude K. McFarland and Karen V. Scipio-Skinner

Patient goals	Nursing interventions	Expected outcomes
Verbalize sexual concerns	Encourage patient to describe current sexual interactions and behavior patterns (e.g., compatibility with sexual partner; comfort with sexual interactions; frequency of sexual interactions) Provide privacy when discussing sexual matters Acknowledge patient's feelings of anxiety about discussing sexual concerns Avoid premature reassurance; provide opportunities for full expression of concerns Provide climate in which patient can openly discuss concerns. Use nonjudgmental attitude	Identifies personal sexual conflicts
Verbalize knowledge about human sexuality	Explore patient's knowledge deficit regarding sexuality (e.g., how did patient learn about sexuality; what is patient's understanding about normal human sexual functions?)	Verbalizes increased knowledge about human sexuality

References: 157, 181, 195, 217, and 261.

Continued.

SEXUAL DYSFUNCTION—cont'd

Patient goals	Nursing interventions	Expected outcomes
	Dispel any myths or misinformation patient may have about sexual activities (e.g., that masturbating will make you crazy)	
	Use terminology that patient understands (e.g., does patient know what the words *coitus* and *sexual intercourse* mean?)	
	Clarify with patient any uncertainties regarding terminology being used (slang or street terminology can have a variety of meanings)	
Identify and discuss personal sexual beliefs and values	Monitor patient's beliefs and values regarding sexuality (How do factors such as patient's early childhood beliefs, religious beliefs, and perception of parental attitudes toward sex affect present beliefs and values?)	Selects socially acceptable behaviors consistent with personal beliefs and values
	Listen to what patient has to say without jumping to conclusions or interpreting behavior prematurely	

Attend closely to verbal and nonverbal signals suggesting anxiety or indications that a problem is more extensive than originally presented

Encourage communications between partners

Recommend a self-help program or refer to individual or group counseling as appropriate

Assist patient in describing behavior rather than labeling (e.g., "I have difficulty becoming sexually aroused" instead of "I am frigid")

Within own scope of knowledge and level of comfort, offer suggestions to patient regarding alternative sexual behaviors or outlets. Allow patient the opportunity to discuss suggestions

Assist patient in determining whether or not a behavior is helpful or useful in reaching goals, instead of labeling behavior as good or bad

Provide specific facts that address expressed needs

Give patient permission to say no or not do something

SEXUALITY PATTERNS, ALTERED

Related factors: Knowledge/skill deficit about alternative responses to health-related transitions; altered body functions or structures; illness or medical treatment.

Carol Kupperberg, Gertrude K. McFarland, and Candice S. Korb

Patient goals	Nursing interventions	Expected outcomes
Attain satisfying level of sexual activity compatible with functional capacity	Provide specific information to patient and partner regarding limitations; correct myths and misinformation Teach patient about possible side effects of drugs such as digitalis, ganglion blocking agents, antidepressants, some hypnotics and tranquilizers, diuretics, alcohol, and beta blockers, as well as other antihypertensive drugs that may affect libido in the woman and may cause decreased libido, difficulty in achieving an erection, and difficulty ejaculating in the man Use premorbid sexual functioning and patterns of sexual activity through sexual history as basis for teaching/counseling	Resumes sexual activity at or near premorbid level at time determined by individual limiting factors

	Address stress, fears, and sexual concerns of partner and examine relationship with sexual partner Examine concerns regarding sexuality and adequacy of sexual function Assess level of comfort in discussing topic alone or with partner; provide opportunity for both Use exercise capability to determine readiness to resume sexual activity (ability to attain a heart rate of 115-120 beats per minute without symptoms) Assist patient in developing individualized plan of progressive physical and sexual activity based on physiological limitations Teach patient to avoid isometric muscular activity to lessen cardiac work load Teach patient that warning signs are increased heart rate and rapid breathing that persists for greater than 15 minutes after intercourse	

References: 1, 298, 415, and 490.

SKIN INTEGRITY, IMPAIRED

Related factors: Physical immobilization; altered circulation.

Kathryn Czurylo and Mi Ja Kim

Patient goals	Nursing interventions	Expected outcomes
Have intact skin in area of disruption	Perform assessment of wound (Stage 1-4) and surrounding skin as a baseline and document regularly Keep skin clean and dry Perform prescribed dressing changes at site of lesion Debride and clean wound as ordered Provide wound treatment (e.g., per order—ointments, plastic coatings, gauze, nonabsorptive thin films, absorptive thick wafers, absorptive gels, enzymatic debriding agents, lubricating spray) Monitor patient closely for signs and symptoms of infection Instruct patient/significant other about the following and have him/her return demonstration: Skin inspection Wound care as ordered Keeping skin clean Skin lubrication	Skin lesion is clean and healing Patient/significant other demonstrates proper skin care

	Protection from environmental agents Skin massage and position changes When to contact physician with problems Signs and symptoms of infection	
Avoid pressure to integument	Keep pressure off lesion Ambulate patient if possible When patient is in bed, turn every 1-2 hours; use all four sides if possible (lateral, prone, dorsal), avoiding positioning on lesion Teach patient to change position if possible Use static devices (foam or water, air, or gel filled) and/or dynamic support systems (air fluidized) as necessary Massage skeletal prominences with lotion every 2 hours Do not massage reddened areas Protect skeletal prominences when positioning with pillows, sheepskin, etc. Prevent HOB elevation greater than 30 degrees for long periods Avoid use of doughnuts, rubber rings	Intact skin around lesion
Maintain circulation to integument	Provide adequate nutrition, including: Increased calories and protein	Healing of lesion: granulation tissue, scar, then intact skin

References: 24, 74, 86, 136, 165, 258, and 450.

Continued.

SKIN INTEGRITY, IMPAIRED—cont'd

Patient goals	Nursing interventions	Expected outcomes
	Fluid intake adequate to prevent dehydration (2600 ml/day if possible) Iron and vitamin C supplements as needed Monitor lab values that impact on skin and report abnormalities: Hct/Hgb Blood glucose BUN Uric acid Albumin Bilirubin Electrolytes ABGs Perform passive ROM every 2 hours to promote circulation to area of lesion	Lab values within normal limits

SKIN INTEGRITY, IMPAIRED, POTENTIAL

Risk factor: Confined to bed rest.

Kathryn Czurylo and Mi Ja Kim

Patient goals	Nursing interventions	Expected outcomes
Maintain intact skin tissue	Keep skin clean and dry after washing Prevent extremes in environmental temperature and humidity Monitor patient for the following risk factors: Mental status Incontinence Immobility Inactivity Poor nutrition Poor hydration Edema Monitor blood chemistry levels that impact on skin and report abnormalities when present: Hct/Hbg Blood glucose	Skin is intact

References: 74, 165, 484, and 487.

Continued.

SKIN INTEGRITY, IMPAIRED, POTENTIAL—cont'd

Patient goals	Nursing interventions	Expected outcomes
	BUN Uric acid Albumin Bilirubin Electrolytes ABGs Instruct patient/significant other about the following and have him/her return demonstration: Skin inspection for redness, cyanosis, blistering, temperature, and pulses Skin cleaning Skin lubrication Protection from environmental agents Skin massage and position changes When to contact physician with problem	
Experience less pressure to integument	Prevent pressure on skin and skeletal prominences as much as possible Ambulate patient if possible	Patient/significant other verbalizes knowledge about proper skin care

	When patient is in bed, turn every 1-2 hours; use all four sides (lateral, prone, dorsal) unless contraindicated Teach patient to change position if possible Use static devices (foam or water, air, or gel filled) as necessary Massage skeletal prominences with lotion every 2 hours Do not massage reddened areas Protect skeletal prominences when positioning with pillows, sheepskin, etc. Prevent HOB elevation greater than 30 degrees for long periods Avoid use of doughnuts, rubber rings	
Maintain adequate circulation to integument	Provide adequate nutrition, including: Sufficient calories and protein Fluid intake adequate to prevent dehydration (2600 ml/day if possible) Have patient do active ROM or do passive ROM for patient every 2 hours to promote circulation to skin Elevate legs to prevent edema	Patient/significant other returns demonstration of proper skin care

SLEEP PATTERN DISTURBANCE

Related factors: Anxiety; depression; disruptions in life-style or usual sleep habits due to illness or hospitalization (e.g., frequent monitoring or therapeutic interventions).

Susan Dudas and Mi Ja Kim

Patient goals	Nursing interventions	Expected outcomes
Understand factors contributing to sleep pattern disturbances	Compare patient's current sleep pattern with usual sleep habits prior to hospitalization Monitor for factors that interfere with sleep (e.g., anxiety, worries) Confer with family/significant others about potential causes of sleep pattern disturbances Discuss possible causes for disturbed sleep (e.g., patient's worries, concerns, pain) Encourage expression of concerns if and when patient is unable to sleep Evaluate effects of patient's medications that may interfere with sleep (e.g., steroids, diuretics) Observe and monitor patient's daytime habits/activities Plan daytime activities	Potential causes for inadequate sleep are determined Specific plan developed to manage or correct causes of inadequate sleep

	Discourage daytime napping *only* if daytime naps negatively affect nighttime sleep Monitor patient in order to avoid excessive time in bed (when possible)	
Fall asleep within 1 hour of going to bed	Provide patient with comfortable environment to promote sleep or rest (i.e., turn off lights, avoid noise disturbances, provide adequate room ventilation, provide warmth or coolness as needed) Promote relaxation at bedtime: select interventions approved by patient (i.e., provide soft music; provide back massage; suggest guided imagery techniques; teach relaxation techniques) Determine patient's usual nighttime habits and provide for routine as closely as possible (e.g., provide warm milk if allowed on regimen and if no nighttime voiding problem exists) Decrease fluid intake prior to bedtime Avoid caffeine for 4 hours before sleep (if fluids are needed, substitute decaffeinated drinks) Have patient empty bladder at bedtime	Patient falls asleep within 1 hour of going to bed Patient acknowledges promptness in falling asleep

References: 143, 185, 186, 216, 379, 422, and 424.

Continued.

SLEEP PATTERN DISTURBANCE—cont'd

Patient goals	Nursing interventions	Expected outcomes
	Avoid strenuous physical or mental activity just before bedtime	
Sleep through the night or at least for increased lengths of uninterrupted periods	Schedule assessments or interventions to allow for longer sleep periods (e.g., check vital signs and turn patient at same time) Help patient to maintain a normal day/night pattern to facilitate night sleeping Provide sedation as prescribed, if necessary Determine effectiveness of sedatives prescribed (i.e., optimal dosage, no rebound effects) Monitor level of daytime alertness	Minimum number of essential interruptions will occur Patient will sleep during longer intervals between nursing care functions Patient will verbalize feeling of being rested or refreshed

SOCIAL INTERACTION, IMPAIRED

Related factors: Knowledge/skill deficit about ways to enhance mutuality; self-concept disturbance; absence of available significant others.

Mary E. Markert and Gertrude K. McFarland

Patient goals	Nursing interventions	Expected outcomes
Express feelings in socially acceptable ways	Use one-to-one relationship Observe for cues (e.g., anxiety level) that patient can tolerate interaction Employ brief contacts at frequent intervals Do not personalize silence, hostile remarks, physical withdrawal from interactions, or rejection of initial attempts to establish relationship Discuss neutral topics or subjects in which patient has an interest Provide opportunities for meaningful task performance within the milieu Give immediate positive feedback for specific behaviors indicative of improvement Demonstrate a caring attitude about patient's feelings and experiences	Demonstrates increased ability to cope with interpersonal encounters and social situations Expresses feelings in a socially acceptable manner

References: 26, 235, 271, 320, 397, 439, and 446.

Continued.

SOCIAL INTERACTION, IMPAIRED—cont'd

Patient goals	Nursing interventions	Expected outcomes
Increase interactions with staff and peers to strengthen ability to relate to others	Use assessment of patient's strengths and capabilities to promote successful interaction Emphasize reality-based conversation and orientation to the present Facilitate conversation between peers Provide time alone, particularly if environmental design does not provide opportunity for solitude Encourage patient to express feelings in ways that seem comfortable but set limits on acting-out behaviors Help patient to identify persons with whom he/she feels comfortable and encourage interactions and activities with them Elicit expressed preferences for roommate, activities, etc. Structure milieu to promote socialization—small areas for reading, activity, etc.	Demonstrates increased ability to cope with interpersonal encounters and social situations

	Provide choices (wearing apparel, menus, etc.) and a safe, nonrestrictive environment Encourage strategies to increase socialization for patients followed in outpatient setting (interaction with family and friends) Help patient to identify situations in which others are alienated because of patient's behaviors related to fears of rejection Avoid excessive stimulation, fright, or discomfort related to increasing demands for interaction or activity Help patient to identify behaviors that may lead to withdrawal into fantasy Steadily reduce amount of idle time Be firm on need for active routine Be flexible, using a neutral or lighthearted approach when encouraging participation in potentially threatening social situations	

Continued.

SOCIAL INTERACTION, IMPAIRED—cont'd

Patient goals	Nursing interventions	Expected outcomes
Engage in normal social activities with individuals and with groups	Help patient move from one-to-one interactions into structured group activities of 4 to 8 persons to perform a task, study a topic, learn a new social skill, etc. Schedule regular group meeting times and facilitate participation by each member Encourage group members to interact with each other and not just with leader Keep group membership stable so that trust, open sharing, and role identification can occur Use creative activities (e.g., painting) to provide opportunity for self-expression and demonstration of talents as well as group interaction When able, encourage increased involvement in community groups (group sports, reading groups, art groups, classes, etc.)	Verbalizes self-perceived change in level of interpersonal confidence

	Practice reciprocal sharing of feelings with discussion of how to set limits and maintain relationships Teach social skills, including the following steps: Help patient identify and clearly define problem Clarify details of problem through pertinent questions Use cognitive skills to organize thoughts, feelings, and behaviors Discuss alternatives and develop a working strategy Observe role models involved in problem situations Role play situations to help patient to experience thought content and process, appropriate affect, and acceptable behavior Identify most appropriate action in light of interpersonal encounter Create a planned program of contact with the community through education and training programs When able, encourage initiative in identifying opportunities for social interaction with friends, family, and community groups	Spends time with family/friends Initiates conversations and focuses on others rather than self Demonstrates principles of effective social relations: Interpersonal complementarity Interpersonal versatility Interpersonal influence

SOCIAL ISOLATION

Related factors: Low self-esteem; arrested psychological development; inability to engage in satisfying personal relationships.

Jane Lancour and Audrey M. McLane

Patient goals	Nursing interventions	Expected outcomes
Develop a trusting relationship	Evaluate social and psychological background Complete measurement of loneliness and self-concept inventory Facilitate and explore expressions of feelings Explore dynamics of past relationships: process and outcome Engage in active listening Maintain open communication Alert patient to negative self-talk and discuss inaccuracies of perception Allow patient to progress at own rate	Demonstrates a trusting relationship by expressing feelings of loneliness, distrust, and sense of self
Reduce degree of social isolation	Give patient information about available, pertinent group therapy Develop plan of action with patient Provide positive reinforcement for even the slightest movement away from pattern of social isolation Structure with patient a self-modification program using strategy of operant conditioning	Spends 1 period per week in group therapy Invites one person to visit home within 2-month period Selects and participates in one leisure group activity every 2 weeks

Develop one or two meaningful relationships	Identify barriers to forming meaningful relationships Discuss relationship of personal responsibility and social isolation Discuss and analyze at each visit positive and negative aspects of interpersonal interactions that occurred in previous week Discuss reality of risks/benefits of opening oneself to others	Identifies two individuals who are important and why they are important Interacts with these individuals on a regular basis
Develop interest in volunteering to assist someone or an organization	Discuss satisfaction that can be experienced through helping others Provide patient with information about volunteer possibilities in immediate vicinity Ask patient to make one phone call per week to obtain information about volunteer services and elicit feelings about that phone call at next session	Makes one phone call per week for 3 weeks, inquiring about volunteer services
Expand and engage in new interests	Negotiate with patient to complete a leisure assessment Explore with patient obstacles to involvement in one leisure activity identified as interesting Help patient to engage in strategies to overcome obstacles	Engages in one satisfying leisure activity appropriate to developmental stage with another individual(s) on a regular basis

References: 107, 355, 359, 388, 390, and 443.

SPIRITUAL DISTRESS (DISTRESS OF THE HUMAN SPIRIT)*

Related factors: Challenged belief in God; separated from formal religious and family support; drug and alcohol abuse; discouraged and apathetic.

Richard J. Fehring and Audrey M. McLane

Patient goals	Nursing interventions	Expected outcomes
Improve spiritual well-being	Provide models of persons who have overcome difficulties, using examples from literature, Bible, personal experiences, etc. Encourage/accept verbalization of feelings of anger Teach cognitive coping strategies (e.g., combating distorted thinking and values clarification) Provide referral to spiritual counselor Monitor spiritual distress with Spiritual Well-Being Index of Paloutzian and Ellison Provide daily prayer/meditation booklet congruent with reading level and expressed religious/denominational preference Use imagery/prayer/music to heal past life hurts	Achieves high score (80-120) on Spiritual Well-Being Index of Paloutzian and Ellison Makes positive statements about self and life Articulates and is comfortable with belief system

Develop support system with friends/church members	Encourage participation in adult prayer, social, and athletic groups Use role playing to prepare patient for new relationships	Initiates ongoing relationship with another individual Feels someone cares about him/her Participates in group activities (alcohol support group, prayer group, etc.)
Participate in alcohol rehabilitation program	Refer and advocate patient's entrance into inpatient alcohol and drug treatment program	Enters and adheres to alcohol rehabilitation program
Find a job and/or engage in volunteer activity	Refer to social worker/vocational counselor Explore volunteer opportunities Enroll in basic reading program	Obtains job counseling Participates in volunteer program Attends basic reading program Articulates goals in life

References: 32, 122, 140, 259, 260, 297, and 352.

*This care plan is for a patient who believes in God and is homeless.

SUFFOCATION, POTENTIAL FOR

Risk factors: Bouts of excessive drinking after ingestion of a large meal; smokes in bed; periodic emesis after drinking.

Audrey M. McLane

Patient goals	Nursing interventions	Expected outcomes
Recognize increased risk of suffocation	Teach patient dangers of smoking in bed	Permanently removes all smoking materials from bedside
	Use anatomic drawings to teach patient/spouse danger of inhaling expelled gastric contents	Establishes a separate area in home for smoking
		Verbalizes understanding of hazards
	Teach spouse to position patient on side to avoid inhaling own vomit	Spouse demonstrates side-lying position and use of supports to keep spouse on side
Participate in alcohol rehabilitation program	Offer patient and spouse opportunity to discuss their perceptions of patient's drinking behavior	Acknowledges drinking problem
	Assist patient in examining consequences of drinking behavior	Verbalizes knowledge of adverse effects of drinking
	Provide patient and spouse with list of alcohol treatment programs	Spouse joins Al-Anon
		Patient enters and adheres to alcohol treatment program

References: 19, 20, and 442.

SWALLOWING, IMPAIRED

Related factors: Decreased gag reflex; decreased strength of muscles involved in mastication; paralysis of left side of face and mouth (4 days post-CVA).

Marilyn Wade, Audrey M. McLane, Linda K. Young, and Marie Maguire

Patient goals	Nursing interventions	Expected outcomes
Maintain adequate nutritional/ hydration status	Provide mouth care before and after meals and dietary supplements Collaborate with dietitian/speech therapist to develop plan for introduction and progression of foods and fluids: Fluid progression: Introduce thick liquids first. Progressively add thin liquids, beginning with juices with most taste (citrus) and most sensation (carbonated beverages). Add thin liquids without much taste last (water, tea, coffee). Always begin with cold liquids and progress to hot Food progression: Introduce foods with pureed consistency first. Progressively add mechanical soft (ground) foods, then solid foods. Begin solid foods with those that require the least chewing	Swallows with assistance of verbal cueing Gradually requires fewer verbal cues to swallow Communicates food preferences (may need to use communication board device)

References: 80, 192, 238, 411, and 445.

Continued.

SWALLOWING, IMPAIRED—cont'd

Patient goals	Nursing interventions	Expected outcomes
	Place foods on unaffected side of mouth Use verbal cueing (name each bite of food, where placed, and when to swallow) Determine food preferences from patient and family members Provide high-calorie nutritional supplement 2 hours after meals and at bedtime Monitor intake (calorie estimates, daily weights) and record I&O	
Improve ability to swallow foods and liquids safely	Follow recommendations of speech therapist to provide consistent approach to facilitate swallowing Position patient upright with head flexed slightly forward at mealtimes to avoid aspiration	Swallows safely without gagging and without aspirating Nonverbal behaviors suggest increased confidence in swallowing ability

	Keep in upright position for ½ hour after eating to prevent aspiration	
	Teach and reinforce with patient/family that swallowing problems may be temporary	
	Praise small gains in ability to swallow	
Have family members participate in care management	Collaborate with speech therapist in teaching swallowing techniques to family members	Family members assist patient with feeding with less supervision over time
	Teach Heimlich maneuver to family members to use in emergency	Family members describe/demonstrate Heimlich maneuver
	Reassure family members about actual/potential improvements in swallowing	Patient/family members make nutritious dietary selections
	Encourage family members to assist patient with selection of nutritious foods	Family members provide encouragement and support during meals
	Establish/maintain private, relaxed atmosphere during meals	

THERMOREGULATION, INEFFECTIVE

Related factor: Immature thermoregulatory system.

Kathryn Czurylo and Mi Ja Kim

Patient goals	Nursing interventions	Expected outcomes
Maintain normothermia	Adjust environmental temperature to patient's needs Adjust patient's temperature, using overhead warmer, warm blankets, or clothing, as necessary During cooling or rewarming, monitor temperature at least every 2 hours Administer IV fluids at room temperature Monitor temperature: axillary every 15 minutes × 4, every 30 minutes × 2, every hour × 4, then every 4 hours, or use continuous monitoring Monitor other vital signs every 15 minutes × 4, every 30 minutes × 2, every hour × 4, then every 4 hours Monitor the following lab values that may be affected by thermal instability: BUN (elevated), serum pH (acidosis), serum electrolytes (hyperkalemia), blood glucose (hypoglycemia) Note and consult physician if signs and symptoms of hypothermia/hyperthermia persist	No signs or symptoms of hypothermia, such as poor feeding, increased or decreased activity, irritability, lethargy, weak cry, tachypnea, tachycardia, grunting, nasal flaring, periods of apnea Temperature: 36° to 36.5° C (skin) 36.5° to 37.5° C (axillary) Other vital signs within normal limits for patient Serum electrolyte and fluid balance within normal limits

References: 310 and 323.

THOUGHT PROCESSES, ALTERED

Related factor: Psychological conflicts.

Evelyn L. Wasli and Gertrude K. McFarland

Patient goals	Nursing interventions	Expected outcomes
Evaluate negative thoughts and feelings and replace with more functional and positive thoughts	Assist patient in identifying specific problem areas Broaden scope of patient's assessment of situation Identify behaviors occurring as result of inaccurate thoughts and note changes needed Assist patient in exploring appropriateness of goal set for self at present time and for the future Work with patient to examine consistency of personal thoughts with basic views of life and values Examine with patient the effects of others, of experts, and of own experience on thoughts Review with patient the usefulness of thoughts in attaining goals or achieving effective relationships Check with patient to see if views are factual	Demonstrates improved self-esteem Expresses more rational thoughts Demonstrates increased problem-solving ability, particularly in examining thoughts, feelings, and behavior relationships Monitors self for negative automatic thoughts Exchanges negative automatic thoughts for positive thought patterning Plans for the future

References: 27, 123, 204, 332, 376, 410, and 413.

Continued.

THOUGHT PROCESSES, ALTERED—cont'd

Patient goals	Nursing interventions	Expected outcomes
	Help patient to learn to watch for own reactions to automatic thoughts Identify stimulus Identify inappropriate response Identify automatic thought Assist patient in identifying cognitive error used most frequently: Associating events occurring relating directly to self or occurring because of self Exaggerating or discounting part or all of own experience	

	Making sweeping generalizations Forming inferences without sufficient data Attending to selected aspects of a situation Applying black and white moral judgments Assist patient in viewing symptoms as cues or signals to take action (i.e., review thoughts, feelings, and behavior) Teach use of techniques such as recording of automatic thoughts, asking another about personal interpretations of situations, rehearsing responses, role playing, using rewards for self, and specific skill training to assist in evaluating and replacing automatic thoughts	

TISSUE INTEGRITY, IMPAIRED

Related factor: Venous pooling.

Mary V. Hanley and Mi Ja Kim

Patient goals	Nursing interventions	Expected outcomes
Maintain tissue perfusion and venous return	Remove constrictive clothing Teach patient to avoid constrictive clothing (e.g., shoes, stockings, tight-waisted undergarments) Demonstrate and assist patient in performing lower-extremity exercises and deep breathing exercises, sequentially, to activate skeletal muscle pump and respiratory pump in lying or standing position Elevate extremity when patient is in sitting position Teach patient to avoid crossing legs Develop an exercise schedule with patient that includes a comfortable combination of walking and rest periods and that avoids standing still for prolonged periods Discontinue smoking Consult with physician if antiembolic stockings are necessary	Edema surrounding lesion is reduced Skin color and temperature are consistent with color and temperature of unaffected extremity Demonstrates and consistently performs circulatory exercises and postural maneuvers

Attain tissue healing	Assess lesion for depth (partial or full thickness) and healing phase (e.g., granulation, epithelialization) Provide physiological and aseptic environment for lesion Clean lesion with nonirritating solutions Remove purulent drainage and necrotic tissue Consult with physician concerning debridement strategies Teach patient to perform wound care and to detect symptoms and signs of infection or increased inflammation Assess dietary intake to determine adequacy of vitamin C and vitamin A, as well as protein Monitor fluid balance (e.g., intake of fluid and salt, urine output, wound drainage [if present], and weight fluctuations)	Wound is free of purulent and necrotic material Demonstrates wound care procedure and describes condition of wound accurately Verbalizes signs and symptoms of inflammation and infection Skin of lower extremity is intact
Reduce oxygen demands	Provide rest periods If patient is overweight, reduce caloric intake to reduce work load to lower extremity	Expresses less fatigue

References: 2, 8, and 60.

TISSUE PERFUSION, ALTERED (PERIPHERAL)

Related factor: Interruption of arterial flow.

Mi Ja Kim and Kathryn Czurylo

Patient goals	Nursing interventions	Expected outcomes
Manifest decreasing signs and symptoms of tissue damage and wound infection	Encourage ambulation if possible Instruct on exercise program or active/passive ROM to extremities every 2 hours as appropriate Keep legs level with or lower than heart Avoid prolonged exposure to cold environmental temperature; room temperature should be 22.2° C-23.3° C Avoid pressure on extremities by use of: Sheepskins Egg crates Heal protectors Water mattress Foot cradle Avoid injury to extremities by teaching patient to: Wear protective shoes Provide good foot care	Improvement or maintenance of peripheral circulation as evidenced by decreased claudication, warmth and good color of extremities, no ulcers Patient/significant other verbalizes knowledge of therapeutic measures Patient/significant other returns demonstration of therapeutic measures if appropriate

	Avoid rubbing or scratching Avoid using hot water bottles or heating pads Teach patient to avoid things that may cause lack of blood flow: Crossing legs Stress Wearing tight clothing Use of knee gatch	
Experience less pain	Administer and teach patient about pain medication and vasodilators as ordered Assist patient in controlling risk factors: Hypertension Smoking High-fat, high-sodium diet Instruct patient about signs and symptoms to report to physician Instruct patient/significant other on above interventions and have him/her do return demonstrations if appropriate	Verbalize less pain

References: 42, 189, 452, and 473.

TRAUMA, POTENTIAL FOR (FALLING)

Risk factors: Unanchored rugs, cluttered hallways, impaired mobility.

Audrey M. McLane

Patient goals	Nursing interventions	Expected outcomes
Adapt home environment to reduce risk of falling	Assist patient in examining hazards in environment	Permanently removes all unanchored rugs
	Identify with patient alternate places to store items in hallways	Hallways are clear and well lighted
	Assist with task of storing items in new locations	
	Develop with patient a list of new storage areas	Keeps an updated list of where items are stored
Increase activity level	Refer patient for free loan of walker from church group	Obtains and uses walker
	Teach patient to walk outdoors with visitors (weather permitting)	Walks outdoors when visitors are willing to provide assistance (e.g., open doors)
	Develop with patient plan to increase walking distance to tolerance level	Increases walking distance 10 ft per week

References: 19, 20, and 442.

UNILATERAL NEGLECT

Related factor: Effects of disturbed perceptual ability related to hemianopsia.

Victoria L. Mock and Gertrude K. McFarland

Patient goals	Nursing interventions	Expected outcomes
Have realistic awareness of perceptual deficit	Explain to patient that one side is being neglected	Verbalizes realistic estimation of degree of deficit—does not ignore or underestimate it
	Encourage patient to share own perception; provide realistic feedback	
Be protected from injury	Provide a safe environment by regularly orienting patient to environment; removing excess furniture and equipment; providing good lighting; placing call bell and frequently used objects on unaffected side within easy reach; keeping side rail up on affected side	Accidents prevented or minimized
	Supervise and/or assist in transferring and ambulating	Absence of injury due to deficit
	Protect neglected side during activities and teach patient to assume this responsibility; teach patient to check position of limbs on affected side to prevent unfelt trauma	
	Note perceptual deficit on patient record and in patient's room to inform caregivers	

References: 40, 164, 351, 380, 460, 489, and 493.

Continued.

UNILATERAL NEGLECT—cont'd

Patient goals	Nursing interventions	Expected outcomes
Acquire knowledge and skill to decrease and/or cope with deficit	Assess regularly for degree of deficit and adaptation to deficit; assess contributing factors Initially, assist compensation for perceptual deficit by arranging environment within patient's perceptual field After initial stress, promote conscious attention to neglected side by placing frequently used items on that side; position patient so that affected side is in view; talk to patient from that side Spend time with patient, manipulating affected side and encouraging patient to use it Have patient handle ignored limbs with unaffected side Increase stimulation to affected side by touching/massage with scented lotion Use visual and verbal communication regarding limb placement on affected side	Responds to verbal and/or visual cues to decrease neglect of affected side; scans and protects affected side Compensates for perceptual loss Demonstrates increased participation and independence in ADLs Verbalizes feeling of progress in regard to perceptual deficit

	Teach patient to scan affected side; place clock or some frequently used item on side of deficit in order to help establish a pattern of scanning	
	Use "cueing" to affected side to increase awareness of that side (e.g., place red line in margin of books on affected side, small bells on limbs of affected side)	
	Place food tray toward unaffected side; teach patient to rotate plate periodically	
	Encourage patient to perform ADLs such as toothbrushing in front of a mirror; supervise and give feedback	
	Decrease confusing stimuli: avoid relocation; maintain consistency of caregivers and consistent routine for self-care; explain procedures and treatment well in advance	
	Include family in rehabilitation process so that they understand it, support it, and can continue it in home environment	

URINARY ELIMINATION, ALTERED PATTERNS

Related factor: Long-term use of Foley catheter.

Ruth E. McShane and Audrey M. McLane

Patient goals	Nursing interventions	Expected outcomes
Establish a normal pattern of urinary elimination	Collaborate with patient to establish regular voiding schedule Teach/monitor use of Kegel's exercises Encourage fluid intake to 1400 ml per day Suggest patient drink 120 ml cranberry juice per day Teach patient protective skin care	Adheres to established voiding schedule Decrease in number of episodes of involuntary loss of urine to occasional loss Drinks 5 to 6 glasses of water per day Skin in perineal area is clean and dry No redness or discomfort in perineal area
Experience decrease in social isolation	Encourage short visits to friends and relatives Suggest regular use of panty liners Encourage patient to contact employer to discuss eventual return to work	Makes short trips to family member's home Reports increase in self-confidence

References: 125, 141, 299, 349, 408, 409, and 467.

URINARY RETENTION

Related factors: Moderate prostatic hypertrophy; postsurgical pain (bowel resection); minimal activity.

Audrey M. McLane and Ruth E. McShane

Patient goals	Nursing interventions	Expected outcomes
Reestablish usual voiding pattern	Use 100% silicone catheter for indwelling catheter in immediate postoperative period Select appropriate catheter size: Too large of a catheter obstructs seminal ducts and may lead to epididymitis and/or prostatitis; usual size is 16–18 French in male patient. French catheter scale: each gradation = ⅓ mm. Too narrow of a catheter is difficult to insert and permits retrograde extension of bacteria Teach patient to stimulate primitive reflexes to encourage voiding after removal of catheter, including the following methods: stroke lower abdomen or inner thighs; pour warm water over perineum; run water in sink; tap over symphysis pubis	Voids every 3 to 4 hours Empties bladder completely Uses Credé maneuver to facilitate complete emptying of bladder (with physician approval)

References: 152, 226, 227, 274, 284, and 467.

Continued.

URINARY RETENTION—cont'd

Patient goals	Nursing interventions	Expected outcomes
Has no signs or symptoms of infection after removal of catheter	Monitor patient for signs and symptoms of urinary tract infection Obtain daily urinalysis if catheter remains in for more than 48 hours Obtain midstream voided specimen 24 hours after removal of catheter and/or with any signs/symptoms of urinary tract infection (e.g., burning, frequency, urge incontinence) Instruct patient/family to call physician if signs/symptoms of infection develop after discharge from hospital	Reports absence of burning, frequency, and urgency Urinalysis confirms absence of infection

Develop/adhere to health practices to prevent urinary infection	Maintain patient's oral/IV intake at 2000 to 2500 ml unless contraindicated Teach patient/family to maintain acid urine (e.g., use superphysiological amounts of ascorbic acid; drink large quantities of cranberry juice)	Takes superphysiological amounts of vitamin C Maintains adequate oral intake by taking 8 oz of fluid with meals, between meals, and in early evening
Increase level of activity	Collaborate with patient to establish increasing activity schedule Provide pain medication ½ hour before walking and initial voiding attempts after removal of catheter Have patient stand to void or walk to bathroom after removal of catheter	Walks with assistance 4 to 5 times a day Requests pain medication ½ hour prior to walking Stands to void or walks to bathroom after removal of catheter

References: 152, 226, 227, 274, 284, and 467.

VIOLENCE, POTENTIAL FOR: SELF-DIRECTED OR DIRECTED AT OTHERS

Risk factor: Toxic reactions to medication; history of violence.

Gertrude K. McFarland and Lorna A. Larson

Patient goals	Nursing interventions	Expected outcomes
Experience a reduced potential for violence	Monitor patient for: Verbal aggression (e.g., angry shouting) Physical aggression against self (e.g., suicidal gestures) Perceptions of self and environment Value system in which violence is viewed as acceptable response Need to defend personal honor Preconceived plan for harming self or others Strong interest in and/or availability of weapons Ideas of persecution Short attention span Low tolerance to frustration Variations in perception Effects of medications Abnormal vital signs Determine additional risk factors: History of physical aggression against objects History of physical aggression against others	Verbalizes less aggression Demonstrates constructive behavior Absence of assaultive behavior Verbalizes anger appropriately Demonstrates positive regard for others Appears in control of behavior Body relaxed and exhibiting normal muscle tension Refrains from harming self or others Laboratory reports within normal limits Identifies approaching loss of self-control and takes action to regain control Refrains from excessive use of sugar, tobacco, and caffeinated drinks Identifies therapeutic resources available to help change behavior (in order to prevent onset of violence) Vital signs are within normal limits for patient

	History of life stressors History of family violence History of parental discipline patterns as child (the more abusive, the greater the potential for violence) Create ward environment that is light, open, and uncrowded with a low noise level with adequate staffing Avoid a tone of voice that suggests nagging, indifference, or pessimism Always respond to questions asked by patient Do not respond to abusive language with abusive language and do not personalize anger Avoid direct confrontation Avoid extensive eye-to-eye contact, especially when anger is intensifying Establish ward norm against physical harm to self or others with set sanctions for infractions Provide one-to-one supportive counseling to assist patient in identifying coping mechanisms	Demonstrates constructive coping skills in dealing with stress and frustration

References: 119, 251, 451, and 496.

Continued.

VIOLENCE, POTENTIAL FOR: SELF-DIRECTED OR DIRECTED AT OTHERS—cont'd

Patient goals	Nursing interventions	Expected outcomes
	Teach alternate coping mechanisms such as negotiating skills, socially acceptable ways of expressing feelings of anger and hostility, and/or stress-reducing/relaxation skills Provide aerobic exercises 30 minutes 3 to 7 times a week Provide one-to-one supportive counseling to recognize consequences of nonadaptive behavior Provide nurse-group psychotherapy to eliminate interpersonal dysfunctions, develop better communication skills, and foster socialization	

Recommend or provide family therapy to increase ego separation, increase the family's ability to let go, and resolve family issues and conflicts

Teach patient that he/she will be held accountable for own behavior (e.g., a patient who breaks something must pay for it or work to pay it off; if injury to self or others occurs, patient must provide restitution within limits of program)

Teach patient to recognize adverse reactions leading to violence that may result from use of certain drugs for treatment

Teach patient to recognize impending violence and to assume responsibility for aborting violent episode

Glossary

ABC[4] PRN REST For Health* Acronym to assist nurses in remembering assessment categories: *A*, activity/rest; *B*, beliefs/decision making, *C*[1], cardiopulmonary; *C*[2], comfort; *C*[3], cognitive/perceptual; *C*[4], communicating; *P*, physical integrity; *R*, role/relationship; *N*, nutrition; *R*, resource management; *E*, elimination; *S*, sensory/motor; *T*, thermoregulation; *F*, feeling; and *H*, host defense.

defining characteristics Signs and symptoms indicating the presence of a nursing diagnosis.

diagnosis qualifier Descriptors used to specify the status of a diagnosis, such as acuity and severity.

diagnostic label Terminology used to name/label a nursing diagnosis

etiology Previous term for related factors.

expected outcomes Changes in patient behaviors resulting from nursing interventions.

functional health pattern Health patterns used for assessment of human functioning.

NANDA North American Nursing Diagnosis Association.

nursing diagnosis† A clinical judgment about an individual, family, or community that is derived through a deliberate, systematic process of data collection and analysis. It provides the basis for prescriptions for definitive therapy for which

---

*Developed by Kim, McFarland, and McLane.

†From Shoemaker JK: Essential features of a nursing diagnosis. In Kim MJ, McFarland GK, and McLane AM, eds: Classification of nursing diagnoses: proceedings of the Fifth National Conference, St Louis, 1984, The CV Mosby Co, p 109.

the nurse is accountable. It is expressed concisely, and it includes the etiology of the condition when known.

patient goals Goals the patient will achieve or achieve in part as a result of nursing interventions.

related factors Factors contributing to an *actual* nursing diagnosis.

risk factors Predisposing factors that increase vulnerability to the development of a nursing diagnosis (used with *potential* nursing diagnoses).

signs and symptoms Objective manifestations and subjective sensation, including perception and feelings.

taxonomy The science of classification (i.e., the study of the general principles of scientific classification).

taxonomy I revised NANDA taxonomy that includes nursing diagnoses newly approved at the Eighth National Conference (1988).

unitary person* "A four-dimensional energy field identified by pattern and organization and manifesting characteristics and behaviors which are different from those of the parts and which cannot be predicted from knowledge of the parts."

validation Verification of data, which may include assessment factors or nursing interventions.

---

*From Kim MJ and Moritz DA: Classification of nursing diagnoses: proceedings of the Third and Fourth National Conferences, St. Louis, 1982, McGraw-Hill Book Co, p 217.

APPENDIX A

Classification of nursing diagnoses by ABC^4 PRN REST For Health

Activity/rest

Activity intolerance
Activity intolerance, potential
Diversional activity deficit
Fatigue
Self-care deficit, bathing/hygiene
Self-care deficit, dressing/grooming
Self-care deficit, feeding
Self-care deficit, toileting
Sleep pattern disturbance

Beliefs/decision making

Adjustment, impaired
Coping, ineffective individual
Decisional conflict (specify)
Health maintenance, altered
Health-seeking behaviors (specify)
Noncompliance (specify)
Spiritual distress (distress of the human spirit)

Cardiopulmonary

Airway clearance, ineffective
Aspiration, potential for
Breathing pattern, ineffective
Cardiac output, decreased
Fluid volume deficit (1)
Fluid volume deficit (2)
Fluid volume deficit, potential
Fluid volume excess
Gas exchange, impaired
Tissue perfusion, altered (specify type) (renal, cerebral, cardiopulmonary, gastrointestinal, peripheral)

Comfort
Pain
Pain, chronic
Cognitive/perceptual
Body image disturbance
Coping, defensive
Denial, ineffective
Knowledge deficit (specify)
Personal identity disturbance
Self-esteem disturbance
Self-esteem, chronic low
Self-esteem, situational low
Thought processes, altered
Communicating
Communication, impaired verbal
Physical integrity
Injury, potential for
Oral mucous membrane, altered
Poisoning, potential for
Skin integrity, impaired
Skin integrity, impaired, potential
Suffocation, potential for
Tissue integrity, impaired
Trauma, potential for
Role/relationship
Coping, family: potential for growth
Coping, ineffective family: compromised
Coping, ineffective family: disabling
Family processes, altered
Growth and development, altered
Parental role conflict
Parenting, altered
Parenting, altered, potential
Rape-trauma syndrome
Rape-trauma syndrome: compound reaction
Rape-trauma syndrome: silent reaction
Role performance, altered
Sexual dysfunction
Sexuality patterns, altered
Social interaction, impaired
Social isolation
Nutrition
Breastfeeding, ineffective
Nutrition, altered: less than body requirements

Nutrition, altered: more than body requirements
Nutrition, altered: potential for more than body requirements
Resource management
Home maintenance management, impaired
Elimination
Bowel incontinence
Constipation
Constipation, colonic
Constipation, perceived
Diarrhea
Incontinence, functional
Incontinence, reflex
Incontinence, stress
Incontinence, total
Incontinence, urge
Urinary elimination, altered patterns
Urinary retention
Sensory/motor
Disuse syndrome, potential for
Dysreflexia
Mobility, impaired physical
Sensory/perceptual alterations (specify) (visual, auditory, kinesthetic, gustatory, tactile, olfactory)
Swallowing, impaired
Unilateral neglect
Thermoregulation
Body temperature, altered, potential
Hyperthermia
Hypothermia
Thermoregulation, ineffective
Feeling
Anxiety
Fear
Grieving, anticipatory
Grieving, dysfunctional
Hopelessness
Post-trauma response
Powerlessness
Violence, potential for: self-directed or directed at others
Host/defense
Infection, potential for

APPENDIX B

Classification of nursing diagnoses by human response patterns (NANDA Taxonomy I—revised)

Exchanging

Altered nutrition: more than body requirements
Altered nutrition: less than body requirements
Altered nutrition: potential for more than body requirements
Potential for infection
Potential altered body temperature
Hypothermia
Hyperthermia
Ineffective thermoregulation
Dysreflexia
Constipation
Perceived constipation
Colonic constipation
Diarrhea
Bowel incontinence
Altered patterns of urinary elimination
Stress incontinence
Reflex incontinence
Urge incontinence
Functional incontinence
Total incontinence
Urinary retention
Altered (specify type) tissue perfusion (renal, cerebral, cardiopulmonary, gastrointestinal, peripheral)
Fluid volume excess
Fluid volume deficit (1)
Fluid volume deficit (2)

Potential fluid volume deficit
Decreased cardiac output
Impaired gas exchange
Ineffective airway clearance
Ineffective breathing pattern
Potential for injury
Potential for suffocation
Potential for poisoning
Potential for trauma
Potential for aspiration
Potential for disuse syndrome
Impaired tissue integrity
Altered oral mucous membrane
Impaired skin integrity
Potential impaired skin integrity

Communicating

Impaired verbal communication

Relating

Impaired social interaction
Social isolation
Altered role performance
Altered parenting
Potential altered parenting
Sexual dysfunction
Altered family processes
Parental role conflict
Altered sexuality patterns

Valuing

Spiritual distress (distress of the human spirit)

Choosing

Ineffective individual coping
Impaired adjustment
Defensive coping
Ineffective denial
Ineffective family coping: disabling
Ineffective family coping: compromised
Family coping: potential for growth
Noncompliance (specify)
Decisional conflict (specify)
Health-seeking behaviors (specify)

Moving

Impaired physical mobility
Activity intolerance
Fatigue

Potential activity intolerance
Sleep pattern disturbance
Diversional activity deficit
Impaired home maintenance management
Altered health maintenance
Feeding self-care deficit
Impaired swallowing
Ineffective breastfeeding
Bathing/hygiene self-care deficit
Dressing/grooming self-care deficit
Toileting self-care deficit
Altered growth and development

Perceiving

Body image disturbance
Self-esteem disturbance
Chronic low self-esteem
Situational low self-esteem
Personal identity disturbance
Sensory/perceptual alterations (specify) (visual, auditory, kinesthetic, gustatory, tactile, olfactory)
Unilateral neglect
Hopelessness
Powerlessness

Knowing

Knowledge deficit (specify)
Altered thought processes

Feeling

Pain
Chronic pain
Dysfunctional grieving
Anticipatory grieving
Potential for violence: self-directed or directed at others
Post-trauma response
Rape-trauma syndrome
Rape-trauma syndrome: compound reaction
Rape-trauma syndrome: silent reaction
Anxiety
Fear

APPENDIX C

Classification of nursing diagnoses by functional health patterns

I. Health perception–health management pattern

Altered health maintenance
Noncompliance (specify)
Potential for infection
Potential for injury
Potential for trauma
Potential for poisoning
Potential for suffocation
Health-seeking behaviors (specify)

II. Nutritional–metabolic pattern

Altered nutrition: potential for more than body requirements
Altered nutrition: more than body requirements
Altered nutrition: less than body requirements
Ineffective breastfeeding
Potential for aspiration
Impaired swallowing
Altered oral mucous membrane
Potential fluid volume deficit
Fluid volume deficit (1)
Fluid volume deficit (2)
Fluid volume excess
Potential impaired skin integrity
Impaired skin integrity
Impaired tissue integrity
Potential altered body temperature
Ineffective thermoregulation
Hyperthermia
Hypothermia

Based on Gordon M: Manual of nursing diagnoses, 1988-1989, St Louis, 1989, The CV Mosby Co.

III. Elimination pattern

Constipation
Perceived constipation
Colonic constipation
Diarrhea
Bowel incontinence
Altered patterns of urinary elimination
Functional incontinence
Reflex incontinence
Stress incontinence
Urge incontinence
Total incontinence
Urinary retention

IV. Activity–exercise pattern

Potential activity intolerance
Activity intolerance
Impaired physical mobility
Potential for disuse syndrome
Fatigue
Bathing/hygiene self-care deficit
Dressing/grooming self-care deficit
Feeding self-care deficit
Toileting self-care deficit
Diversional activity deficit
Impaired home maintenance management
Ineffective airway clearance
Ineffective breathing pattern
Impaired gas exchange
Decreased cardiac output
Altered (specify type) tissue perfusion (renal, cerebral, cardiopulmonary, gastrointestinal, peripheral)
Dysreflexia
Altered growth and development

V. Sleep–rest pattern

Sleep pattern disturbance

VI. Cognitive–perceptual pattern

Pain
Chronic pain
Sensory perceptual alterations (specify) (visual, auditory, kinesthetic, gustatory, tactile, olfactory)
Unilateral neglect
Knowledge deficit (specify)
Altered thought processes
Decisional conflict (specify)

VII. Self-perception–self-concept pattern

Fear
Anxiety
Hopelessness
Powerlessness
Body image disturbance
Personal identity disturbance
Self-esteem disturbance
Chronic low self-esteem
Situational low self-esteem

VIII. Role–relationship pattern

Anticipatory grieving
Dysfunctional grieving
Altered role performance
Social isolation
Impaired social interaction
Altered family processes
Potential altered parenting
Altered parenting
Parental role conflict
Impaired verbal communication
Potential for violence: self-directed or directed at others

IX. Sexuality–reproductive pattern

Sexual dysfunction
Altered sexuality patterns
Rape-trauma syndrome
Rape-trauma syndrome: compound reaction
Rape-trauma syndrome: silent reaction

X. Coping–stress tolerance pattern

Ineffective individual coping
Defensive coping
Ineffective denial
Impaired adjustment
Post-trauma response
Family coping: potential for growth
Ineffective family coping: compromised
Ineffective family coping: disabling

XI. Value–belief pattern

Spiritual distress (distress of the human spirit)

REFERENCES

1. Abbott MA and McWhirter DP: Resuming sexual activity after myocardial infarction, Med Asp Hum Sex 12(6):18-28, 1978.
2. Abruzzese R, ed: The integumentary system, Top Clin Nurs 5(2), 1983.
3. Ackerman M: The use of bolus normal saline instillations in artificial airways: is it useful or necessary? Heart Lung 14(5):505-506, 1985.
4. Affleck JW and McGuire RJ: The measurement of psychiatric rehabilitation status: a review of the needs and a new scale, Br J Psychiatry 145:517-525, 1984.
5. Alexander HE, McCarty K, and Giffen MB: Hypotension and cardiopulmonary arrest associated with concurrent haloperidol and propranolol therapy, JAMA 252(1):87-88, 1984.
6. Allan JD: Exercise program. In Bulechek GM and McCloskey JC, eds: Nursing interventions: treatments for nursing diagnoses, Philadelphia, 1985, WB Saunders Co.
7. Allen HA, Halparin J, and Friend R: Removal and diversion tactics and the control of auditory hallucinations, Behav Res Ther 5:601-605, 1985.
8. Alterescu KB and Alterescu V: The treatment of pressure sores. In Catania PN and Rosner MM, eds: Home health care practice, Palo Alto, Calif, 1986, Health Markets Research.
9. American Nurses Association and Arthritis Health Professionals Association: Outcome standards for rheumatology nursing practice, Kansas City, Mo, 1983, American Nurses Association.
10. Anderson GH and Hrboticky N: Approaches to assessing the dietary component of the diet-behavior connection, Nutr Rev Suppl, pp 42-50, May 1986.
11. Anderson JM: The social construction of illness experience: families with a chronically ill child, J Adv Nurs 6:427-432, 1981.
12. Anderson JZ and White GD: An empirical investigation of interaction and relationship patterns in functional and dysfunctional nuclear families and stepfamilies, Fam Process 25:407-422, 1986.
13. Andreoli KG, Zipes DP, Wallace AG, Kinney MR, and Fowkes VK: Comprehensive cardiac care, ed 6, St Louis, 1986, The CV Mosby Co.
14. Andrews H and Roy C: Essentials of the Roy Adaptation Model, Norwalk, Conn, 1986, Appleton-Century-Crofts.
15. Anman B: Home care for the high risk infant: a holistic guide to using technology, Rockville, Md, 1986, Aspen Publishers, Inc.
16. Annon JS: Behavioral treatment of sexual problems: brief therapy, Hagerstown, Md, 1976, Harper & Row, Publishers, Inc.
17. Autry D, Lauzon F, and Holliday P: The voiding record: an aid in decreasing incontinence, Geriatr Nurs 5(1):22-25, 1984.
18. Baer CA, Delorey M, and Fitzmaurice JB: A study to evaluate the validity of the rating system for self-care deficit. In Kim MJ, McFarland GK, and McLane AM, eds: Classification of nursing

diagnoses: proceedings of the Fifth National Conference, St Louis, 1984, The CV Mosby Co.
19. Baker S and Dietz P: Injury prevention. In Healthy people, the Surgeon General's report on health promotion and disease prevention: background papers, DHEW-PHS Pub No 79-55071A, Washington, DC, 1979, US Government Printing Office.
20. Baker S, O'Neill B and Karpf R: The injury fact book, Lexington, Mass, 1984, DC Heath & Co.
21. Baker WL and Smith SL: Pulmonary aspiration and tube feedings: nursing implications, Focus Crit Care 11(2):25-27, 1984.
22. Barker WF: Peripheral arterial disease, ed 2, Philadelphia, 1975, WB Saunders Co.
23. Barnes C and Kirchhoff KT: Minimizing hypoxemia due to endotracheal suctioning: a review of the literature, Heart Lung 15(2):164-176, 1986.
24. Barnes S: Patient/family education for the patient with a pressure necrosis, Nurs Clin North Am 22(2):463-474, 1987.
25. Battle EH and Hanna CE: Evaluation of a dietary regimen for chronic constipation: report of a pilot study, J Gerontol Nurs 6:527-532, 1980.
26. Beard M, Enlow C, and Owens J: Activity therapy as a reconstructive plan on the social competence of chronic hospitalized patients, J Psychiatr Nurs Ment Health Serv 16:33-41, Feb 1978.
27. Beck AT: Cognitive therapy. In Kaplan HI and Sadock BJ, eds: Comprehensive textbook of psychiatry, IV, vol 2, Baltimore, 1985, Williams & Wilkins.
28. Beck AT, Rush AJ, and Shaw N: Cognitive therapy of depression, New York, 1979, The Guilford Press.
29. Beck S: Impact of a systemic oral care protocol on stomatitis after chemotherapy, Cancer Nurs 2(3):185-199, 1979.
30. Beglinger JE: Coping tasks in critical care, Dimens Crit Care Nurs 2(2):80-89, 1983.
31. Bellemare F and Grassino A: Force reserve of the diaphragm in patients with chronic obstructive pulmonary disease, J Appl Physiol 55:8-15, 1983.
32. Benson H and Proctor W: Beyond the relaxation response, New York, 1984, Berkley Publishing Group.
33. Bentall RP and Slade PD: Reality testing and auditory hallucinations: a signal detection analysis, Br J Clin Psychol 24(PT3):159-169, Sept 1985.
34. Beske EJ and Garvis MS: Important factors in breastfeeding success, MCN 7:174-179, 1982.
35. Biddle CJ and Biddle WL: A plastic head cover to reduce surgical heat loss, Geriatr Nurs 6(1):39-41, 1985.
36. Blackburn GL, Bistrian BR, Maini BS, Schlamm HT, and Smith MF: Nutritional and metabolic assessment of the hospitalized patient, J Parenteral Enteral Nutr 1:11-22, 1977.
37. Bond JH: Office-based management of diarrhea, Geriatrics 37:52-64, 1982.

38. Bonica JJ: The need for a taxonomy of pain, Pain 6(3):247-249, 1979.
39. Boogaard MAK: Rehabilitation of the female patient after myocardial infarction, Nurs Clin North Am 19:433, 1984.
40. Booth K: The neglect syndrome, J Neurosurg Nurs 14(1):38-43, 1982.
41. Boozer M and Craven R: Nursing strategies for common vascular problems: nursing diagnosis, interventions, evaluation. In Patrick M, Woods S, Craven R, Rokosky J, and Bruno P, eds: Medical-surgical nursing: pathophysiological concepts, Philadelphia, 1986, JB Lippincott Co.
42. Boozer M et al: Nursing care of the patient with chronic occlusive peripheral artery disease. Cardiovasc Nurs 15:13, July 1981.
43. Bowers S and Marshall L: Severe head injury: current treatment and research, J Neurosurg Nurs 14:210-219, Oct 1982.
44. Bowie DM, LeBlanc P, Killian KG, Summers E, and Jones NL: Can the intensity of breathlessness be predicted from the inspiratory flow rate? Am Rev Respir Dis 129A:239, 1984.
45. Bozian MW: Nutrition for the aged or aged nutrition? Nurs Clin North Am 11:169-177, 1976.
46. Brady JP: Social skills training for psychiatric patients. I. Concepts, methods, and clinical results, Am J Psychiatry 141(3):333-340, 1984.
47. Brady JP: Social skills training for psychiatric patients. II. Clinical outcome studies, Am J Psychiatry 141(4):491-498, 1984.
48. Brager B and Yasko J: Stomatitis, in care of the client receiving chemotherapy, Reston, Va, 1984, Reston Publishing Co, Inc.
49. Brandstetter RD, Zakkay Y, Gutherz P, and Goldberg R: Effect of nasogastric feedings on arterial oxygen tension in patients with symptomatic chronic obstructive pulmonary disease, Heart Lung 17(2):170-172, 1988.
50. Brandt PA and Weinert C: The PRQ: a social support measure, Nurs Res 30:277-280, 1981.
51. Braun SR, Dixon RM, Keim NL, Luby M, Anderegg A, and Shrago ES: Predictive clinical value of nutritional assessment factors in COPD, Chest 85:353-357, 1984.
52. Braunwald E: Regulation of the circulation, N Engl J Med 290:1124, 1974.
53. Breslin EH and Lery MJ: Prevention and treatment of aspiration pneumonitis secondary to massive gastric aspiration, Crit Care Q, pp 73-83, 1983.
54. Brewerton TD, Heffernan MM, and Rosenthal NE: Psychiatric aspects of the relationship between eating and mood, Nutr Rev Suppl, pp 78-88, May 1986.
55. Breznitz S: The seven kinds of denial. In Breznitz S, ed: The denial of stress, New York, 1983, International Universities Press, Inc.
56. Brocklehurst JC: How to define and treat constipation, Geriatrics, pp 85-87, June 1977.

57. Brown N, Muhlenkowp A, Fox L, and Osborn M: The relationship among health beliefs, health values, and health promotion activity, West J Nurs Res 5:155-163, 1983.
58. Brunner LS and Suddarth DS: Textbook of medical-surgical nursing, Philadelphia, 1984, JB Lippincott Co.
59. Brunner LS and Suddarth DS: Lippincott manual of nursing practice, Philadelphia, 1986, JB Lippincott Co.
60. Bruno P: Injury: inflammatory response and resolution. In Patrick M, Woods S, Craven R, Rokosky J, and Bruno P, eds: Medical-surgical nursing: pathophysiological concepts, Philadelphia, 1986, JB Lippincott Co.
61. Bulechek GM and McCloskey JC, eds: Nursing interventions: treatments for nursing diagnoses, Philadelphia, 1985, WB Saunders Co.
62. Burckhardt CS: Coping strategies of the chronically ill, Nurs Clin North Am 22(3):543-550, 1987.
63. Burgess AW and Holstrom LL: Rape trauma syndrome, Am J Psychiatry 131:981-986, 1974.
64. Burgess AW and Holstrom LL: Rape: sexual disruption and recovery, Am J Orthopsychiatry 49:648-657, 1979.
65. Burgio KL: A continence clinic: using biofeedback and other behavioral methods for the treatment of urinary incontinence. Paper presentation, CNR Conference: Nursing research: integration into the social structure, San Diego, 1985.
66. Burgio KL, Whitehead WE, and Engel BT: Urinary incontinence in the elderly: bladder-sphincter biofeedback and toilet skills training, Ann Intern Med 104:507-515, 1984.
67. Burns DD: Feeling good: the new mood therapy, New York, 1981, New American Library.
68. Burr WR, Hill R, Nye FI, and Reiss JL, eds: Contemporary theories about the family, vol I, Research based theories, New York, 1979, Free Press.
69. Carlson AC: Infection prophylaxis in the patient with cancer, Oncol Nurs Forum 12:53-64, 1985.
70. Carlson CE and Blackwell B, eds: Behavioral concepts and nursing interventions, Philadelphia, 1978, JB Lippincott Co.
71. Carpenter KD: Recognizing the many faces of fear, Nurs Life 6(4):29-32, 1986.
72. Carroll SM: Clinical validation study of hypothermia: identification of defining characteristics, Unpublished manuscript.
73. Caspersen CJ, Powell KE, and Christenson GM: Physical activity, exercise, and physical fitness: definitions and distinctions for health-related research, Public Health Rep 100:126-146, 1985.
74. Chagares R and Jackson B: How six pressure-relieving devices stack up, Am J Nurs 87(2):191-193, 1987.
75. Chernoff R and Dean JA: Medical and nutritional aspects of intractable diarrhea, J Am Diet Assoc 76:161-169, 1980.
76. Clarren S: Recognition of fetal alcohol syndrome, JAMA 245(23):2436-2439, 1981.

77. Clay E: Habit retraining: a tested method to regain urinary control, Geriatr Nurs 1:252-254, Dec 1980.
78. Clay E: Urinary continence/incontinence: habit training; a tested method to regain urinary control, Geriatr Nurs 1:252-254, 1980.
79. Clements IM and Buchanan DM, eds: Family therapy: a nursing perspective, New York, 1982, John Wiley & Sons, Inc.
80. Cockcroft G and Ray M: Feeding problems in stroke patients, Nurs Mirror 160(9):26-29, 1985.
81. Cohen CA, Zagelbaum G, Gross D, Roussos C, and Macklem PT: Clinical manifestations of inspiratory muscle fatigue, Am J Med 73:308-316, 1982.
82. Cohen P, Pinching A, Rees A, and Peters D: Infection and immunosuppression, Q J Med 51:1-15, 1982.
83. Cohn J: Vasodilator therapy: implications in acute myocardial infarction and congestive heart failure, Am Heart J 49:45, 1982.
84. Cohn JN et al: Effect of vasodilator therapy on mortality in chronic congestive heart failure, N Engl J Nurs, pp 1547-1551, June 1986.
85. Conn EH, Williams RF, and Wallace AG: Physical conditioning in coronary patients with left ventricular dysfunction. In Wenger NK and Hellerstein HK, eds: Rehabilitation in the coronary patient, ed 2, New York, 1984, John Wiley & Sons, Inc.
86. Cooper D: Pressure ulcers: Unpublished research 1976-1986: Process to outcome, Nurs Clin North Am 22(2):475-402, 1987.
87. Cousins N: The healing heart, New York, 1983, WW Norton & Co.
88. Cox CL, Miller EH, and Mull CS: Motivation in health behavior: measurement, antecedents, and correlates, Adv Nurs Sci 9(4):1-15, 1987.
89. Creason NS, Pogue NJ, Nelson AA, and Hoyt CA: Validating the diagnosis of impaired physical mobility, Nurs Clin North Am 20:669-683, 1985.
90. Crouch MA and Straub V: Enhancement of self-esteem in adults, Fam Community Health 6(2):67-78, 1983.
91. Crumbaugh JC and Maholick LT: Purpose in life test. Available from Psychometric Affiliates, PO Box 3167, Munster, Ind 46231.
92. Daeffler R: Oral hygiene measures for patients with cancer, I, Cancer Nurs 3(5):347-356, 1980.
93. Daeffler R: Oral hygiene measures for patients with cancer, II, Cancer Nurs 3(6):427-432, 1980.
94. Daeffler R: Oral hygiene measures for patients with cancer, III, Cancer Nurs 4(1):29-35, 1981.
95. Darrow G and Anthonisen N: Physiotherapy in hospitalized medical patients, Am Rev Respir Dis 122(5) (part 2):155-158, 1980.
96. Davis M, Eshelman ER, and McKay M: The relaxation and stress reduction workbook, Oakland, Calif, 1982, New Harbinger Publishers.
97. Dean PG: Monitoring an apneic infant: impact on the infant's mother, Matern Child Nurs J 15(2):65-76, 1986.
98. DeCarlo JJ and Mann WC: The effectiveness of verbal versus

activity groups in improving self-perceptions of interpersonal communication skills, Am J Occup Ther 39(1):20-27, 1985.

99. DeCarvalho M, Robertson S, and Klaus MH: Does the duration and frequency of early breastfeeding affect nipple pain? Birth 11(2):81-84, 1984.
100. Denis G, Semenza C, Stoppa E, and Lis A: Unilateral spatial neglect and recovery from hemiplegia, Cortex 105:543-552, 1982.
101. De Young S: The neurologic patient—a nursing perspective, Englewood Cliffs, NJ, 1983, Prentice-Hall.
102. DiMatteo M and DiNicola D: Achieving patient compliance: the psychology of the medical practitioner's role, New York, 1982, Pergamon Press.
103. Dishman RK, Sallis JF, and Orenstein DR: The determinants of physical activity and exercise, Public Health Rep 100:158-171, 1985.
104. DiVasto P: Measuring the aftermath of rape, J Psychosoc Nurs 23:33-35, 1985.
105. Dixon J: Effect of nursing interventions on nutritional and performance status of cancer patients, Nurs Res 33:330-335, 1984.
106. Doe WV and Barr GD: Acute diarrhea in adults, Aust Fam Physician 10:438-446, 1981.
107. Doenges M and Moorhouse M: Nurse's pocket guide: nursing diagnoses with interventions, Philadelphia, 1985, FA Davis Co.
108. Doerr BC and Jones JW: Effects of family preparation on the state anxiety level of the CCU patient, Nurs Res 28:315-316, 1979.
109. Done DJ and Frith CD: The effect of context during ward perception in schizophrenic patients, Brain Lang 23(2):318-336, 1984.
110. Donner GJ: Parenthood as a crisis: a role for the psychiatric nurse, Perspect Psychiatr Care 10:84-87, 1972.
111. Donohue W, Giovannoni R, Goldberg A, Keens T, Make B, Plummer A, and Prentice W: Long term mechanical ventilation: guidelines for management in the home and at alternate community sites, Chest 90(suppl. I):1S-37S, 1986.
112. Dougherty CM: Defining the characteristics and interventions for the nursing diagnosis of decreased cardiac output, a poster presentation on Classification of Nursing Diagnosis, St Louis, 1981.
113. Dracup K and Bren C: Using nursing research findings to meet the needs of grieving spouses, Nurs Res 27:212-216, 1978.
114. Drummond G: Hypothermia: its causes, effects, and treatment in the very young and old, Nurs Times 75:2115-2116, 1979.
115. Dufault A: Urinary incontinence: United States and British nursing perspectives, J Gerontol Nurs, pp 28-33, March-Apr 1978.
116. Dufault KJ and Martocchio B: Hope: its spheres and dimensions, Nurs Clin North Am 20:379-391, 1985.
117. Eastwood HDH and Warrell R: Urinary incontinence in the elderly female: prediction in diagnosis and outcome of management, Age Aging 13:230-234, 1984.

118. Ebersole P and Hess P: Toward healthy aging: human needs and nursing response, St Louis, 1985, The CV Mosby Co.
119. Eichelman B: Toward a rational pharmacotherapy for aggressive and violent behavior, Hosp Community Psychiatry 39(1):31-39, 1988.
120. Engel B: Fecal incontinence and encopresis: a psychophysiological analysis. In Holzi R, ed: Psychophysiology of the gastrointestinal tract, New York, 1983, Plenum Publishing Corp.
121. Erickson R: Thermometer placement for oral temperature measurement in febrile adults, Int J Nurs Stud 13:199-208, 1976.
122. Fehring RJ and McLane AM: Spiritual distress. In Thompson JM, McFarland GK, Hirsch JE, Tucker SM, and Bowers AC, eds: Clinical nursing, St Louis, 1985, The CV Mosby Co.
123. Fennell M and Teasdale JD: Cognitive therapy for depression: individual differences and the process of, Cogn Ther Res 2(2):253-271, 1987.
124. Fibison WJ, ed: Special issue on prenatal diagnosis, Issues Health Care Women 1:1-92.
125. Field MS: Urinary incontinence in the elderly: an overview, J Gerontol Nurs 5:12-19, 1979.
126. Fife BL, Huhman M, and Keck J: Development of a clinical assessment scale: evaluation of the psychosocial impact of childhood illness on the family, Issues Compr Pediatr Nurs 9:11-31, 1986.
127. Fiorello J and Blattner B: Creating health for a new age, Home Healthcare Nurse 2:18-32, 1984.
128. Fitzmaurice JB: Utilization of cues in judgments of activity intolerance. In McLane AM, ed: Classification of nursing diagnoses: proceedings of the Seventh Conference, St Louis, 1987, The CV Mosby Co.
129. Fletcher: Current concepts in the nature and treatment of fever, Physician Assist 11(1):95, 1987.
130. Floyd JA: Interaction between personal sleep-wake rhythms and psychiatric hospital rest-activity schedule, Nurs Res 33(5):255-259, 1984.
131. Forchuk C and Westwell J: Denial, J Psychosoc Nurs 25(6):9-13, 1987.
132. Forese G: Heat losses from the human head, J Appl Physiol 10(12):235-241, 1957.
133. Forsyth GL, Delaney KD, and Gresham ML: Vying for a winning position: management style of the chronically ill, Res Nurs Health, 7:181-188, 1984.
134. Fortinsky RH, Granger CV, and Seltzer GB: The uses of functional assessment in understanding home care needs, Med Care 19:489-497, 1981.
135. Fowler E: Equipment and products used in the management and treatment of pressure ulcers, Nurs Clin North Am 22(2):449-461, 1987.
136. Fowler E and Goupil DL: Comparison of the wet-to-dry dressing

and a copolymer starch in the management of debrided pressure sores, J Enterostomal Ther 11(1):22-25, 1984.
137. Foxall MJ, Ekberg JY, and Griffith N: Comparative study of adjustment patterns of chronic obstructive pulmonary disease patients and peripheral vascular disease patients, Heart Lung 16(4):354-363, 1987.
138. Foy DW, Wallace CJ, and Liberman RP: Advances in social skills training for chronic mental patients. In Craig KD and McMahon RJ, eds: Advances in clinical behavior therapy, New York, 1983, Brunner/Mazel, Inc.
139. Francis B: Hot and cold therapy, J Nurs Care 15(2):18-20, 1982.
140. Frankl V: Man's search for meaning, Boston, 1963, Beacon Press.
141. Freed SL: Urinary incontinence in the elderly, Hosp Pract 17:81-94, 1982.
142. Friedman-Campbell M and Hart CA: Theoretical strategies and nursing interventions to promote psychosocial adaptation to spinal cord injuries and disability, J Neurosurg Nurs 16:335-342, 1984.
143. Fry JM: Sleep disorders, Med Clin North Am 71(1):93-108, 1987.
144. Galinsky E: Between generations: the six stages of parenthood, New York, 1981, Times Books.
145. Gallagher CG, Im Hof V, and Younes M: Effect of inspiratory muscle fatigue on breathing pattern, J Appl Physiol 59:1152-1158, 1985.
146. Gardner G: Home I.V. therapy, I, Nat Intraven Ther Assoc 9:95-103, 1986.
147. Gardner C: Home IV therapy, II, Nat Intraven Ther Assoc 9:193-203, 1986.
148. Geer JH: The development of a scale to measure fear, Behav Res Ther 3:45-53, 1965.
149. Gentry WD, Baider L, Oude-Weme JD, Musch F, and Gary HE: Type A/B difference in coping with acute myocardial infarction: further considerations, Heart Lung 12:212-214, 1983.
150. Gerber RM and Van Ort SR: Topical application of insulin in decubitus ulcers, Nurs Res 28:16-19, 1979.
151. Gerety EH and Caley JM: A nurse led encouragement group for families of terminally ill patients, Unpublished manuscript.
152. Gettrust K, Ryan S, and Engelman DS, eds: Applied nursing diagnosis: guide for comprehensive care planning, New York, 1985, John Wiley & Sons, Inc.
153. Getty C and Humphrys W: Understanding the family: stress and change in American family life, Norwalk, Conn, 1981, Appleton-Century-Crofts.
154. Gilberts R: The evaluation of self-esteem, Fam Community Health 6(2):29-49, 1983.
155. Gilliss L: The family as a unit of analysis: strategies for the nurse researchers, Adv Nurs Sci 5(3):50-59, 1983.
156. Glauser F, Polatty R, and Sessler C: State of the art: worsening oxygenation in the mechanically ventilated patient—causes,

mechanisms, and early detection, Am Rev Respir Dis, 138(2):458-465, 1988.
157. Glover J: Human sexuality in nursing care, New York, 1985, Appleton-Century-Crofts.
158. Goldberg M and Roe C: Temperature changes during anesthesia and operations, Arch Surg 98:365-374, Aug 1966.
159. Goldberg R: Temperature changes; Jones H and McLaren C: Postoperative shivering and hypoxaemic after halothane, nitrous oxide and oxygen anaesthesia, Br J Anaesth 37:35-40, 1965; Stephen C: Post-operative changes, Anesthesiology 22:795-799, Sept-Oct 1961.
160. Goldenberg I and Goldenberg H: Family therapy: an overview, ed 2, Monterey, Calif, 1985, Brooks/Cole Publishing Co.
161. Goldstein N et al: Self-care: a framework for the future. In Chinn PL, ed: Advances in nursing theory development, Rockville, Md, 1983, Aspen Systems Corp.
162. Gordon M: Assessing activity tolerance, Am J Nurs 76(1):72-75, 1976.
163. Gordon VC and Ledray LE: Growth-support intervention for the treatment of depression in women of middle years, West J Nurs Res 8(3):263-283, 1986.
164. Gordon WA, Hibbard MR, Egelko S, Dillar L, Shaver MS, Lieberman A, and Ragnarsson K: Perceptual remediation in patients with right brain damage: a comprehensive program, Arch Phys Med Rehabil, 66:353-359, 1985.
165. Gosnell D: Assessment and evaluation of pressure sores, Nurs Clin North Am 22(2):399-416, 1987.
166. Grandjean E: Fatigue: its physiological and psychological significance, Ergonomics 11(5):427-436, 1988.
167. Groer M and Shekleton M: Basic pathophysiology: a conceptual approach, St Louis, 1983, The CV Mosby Co (Chapter 18: Effects of immobility).
168. Gulick EE: Informational correlates of successful breastfeeding, MCN 7:370-375, 1982.
169. Gurevich I and Tafuro P: Nursing measures for the prevention of infection in the compromised host, Nurs Clin North Am 20(1):257-260, 1985.
170. Habeeb MC and Kallstrom MD: Bowel program for institutionalized adults, Am J Nurs 76:606-608, 1976.
171. Hackett TP, Cassem NH, and Wishnie HA: The coronary-care unit: an appraisal of its psychologic hazards, N Engl J Med 279:1365-1370, 1968.
172. Hallal JC: Mobility, impaired physical. In Thompson JM, McFarland GK, Hirsch JE, Tucker SM, and Bowers AC, eds: Clinical nursing, St Louis, 1985, The CV Mosby Co.
173. Hammond WP: Infections in the compromised host, Hosp Med 19:132, Oct 1983.
174. Hampe S: Needs of the grieving spouse in a hospital setting, Nurs Res 24:113-120, 1975.

175. Hanley MV, Rudd T, and Butler J: What happens to intratracheal saline instillations? Am Rev Respir Dis 117(4, part 2, suppl):124, 1978.
176. Hanley MV and Tyler ML: Ineffective airway clearance related to airway infection, Nurs Clin North Am 22(1):135-150, 1987.
177. Hanson J, Jones K, and Smith D: Fetal alcohol syndrome: experience with 41 patients, JAMA 235(14):1458-1460, 1976.
178. Harbouriew: Anger management program, helping angry and violent people manage their emotions and behavior, Hosp Community Psychiatry 38:1207-1210, 1987.
179. Hartfield MT, Cason CL, and Cason GJ: Effects of information about a threatening procedure on patients' expectations and emotional distress, Nurs Res 31(4):202-206, 1982.
180. Hartman CR and Burgess AW: Pattern 10: sexuality—reproductive. In Thompson JM, McFarland GK, Hirsch JE, Tucker SM, and Bowers AC, eds: Clinical nursing, St Louis, 1986, The CV Mosby Co.
181. Hawton K: Sex therapy: a practical guide, New York, 1985, Oxford University Press.
182. Haylock PJ and Hart LK: Fatigue in patients receiving localized radiation, Cancer Nurs 2(6):461-467, 1979.
183. Haynes RB, Taylor DW, and Sackett HD, eds: Compliance in health care, Baltimore, 1979, The Johns Hopkins University Press.
184. Hayter J: Hypothermia/hyperthermia in older persons, J Gerontol Nurs 6(2):65-68, 1980.
185. Hayter J: Sleep behaviors of older persons, Nurs Res 32(4):242-246, 1983.
186. Hayter-Muncy J: Measures to rid sleeplessness, J Gerontol Nurs 12:6-11, 1986.
187. Heineman HS: What to do for the patient with fever, Consultant 18(6):21-24, 1978.
188. Hennessy K: HHN dehydration, Am J Nurs, pp 1425-1426, Oct 1983.
189. Herman JA: Nursing assessment and nursing diagnosis in patients with peripheral vascular disease, Nurs Clin North Am 21:219-231, 1986.
190. Hewat RJ and Ellis DJ: A comparison of the effectiveness of two methods of nipple care, Birth 14(1):41-45, 1987.
191. Hewitt AL, Longmire WT, and Page CF: Geriatric urology flow charts: urinary incontinence—another bane of aging, Patient Care 14:169-171, 1980.
192. Hickey J: Cerebral vascular accident. In Neurological and neurosurgical nursing, ed 2, Philadelphia, 1986, JB Lippincott Co.
193. Hickey SS: Enabling hope, Cancer Nurs 9:133-137, 1986.
194. Hoff LA: People in crisis: understanding and helping, Toronto, 1978, Addison-Wesley Publishing Co, Inc.
195. Hogan R: Human sexuality: a nursing perceptive, New York, 1980, Appleton-Century-Crofts.

196. Holaday B: Challenges of rearing a chronically ill child: caring and coping, Nurs Clin North Am 12:139-147, 1981.
197. Hoskins L et al: Activity/exercise. In Thompson JM, McFarland GK, Hirsch JE, Tucker SM, and Bowers AC, eds: Clinical nursing, St Louis, 1986, The CV Mosby Co.
198. Hoskins LM et al: Mobility, impaired physical. In Thompson JM, McFarland GK, Hirsch JE, Tucker SM, and Bowers AC, eds: Clinical nursing, St Louis, 1986, The CV Mosby Co.
199. Howard M, Vinod K, and Paidpaty B: The effects of fluid resuscitation in the critically ill patient, Heart Lung 13(6):649-654, 1984.
200. Howard RB and Schnell RR: The psychology of diet and behavior modification. In Howard RB and Herbold NH, eds: Nutrition in clinical care, New York, 1978, McGraw-Hill Book Co.
201. Huang SH et al: Coronary care nursing, Philadelphia, 1983, WB Saunders Co.
202. Huss P et al: The new inotropic drug, Doubutamine, Heart Lung, pp 121-126, Jan-Feb 1981.
203. Hymonovich DP: The chronicity impact and coping instrument: parent questionnaire for use by clinicians and researchers, Nurs Res 32:275-281, 1983.
204. Ingram RE and Kendall PC: The cognitive side of anxiety, Cogn Ther Res 2(5):523-536, 1987.
205. Iveson-Iveson J: Body temperature, Nurs Mirror 154:32, 1982.
206. Jacox A, ed: Pain: a source book for nurses and other health professionals, Boston, 1977, Little, Brown & Co, Inc.
207. James SR and Mott SR: Child health nursing: essential care of children and families, Menlo Park, Calif, 1988, Addison-Wesley Publishing Co, Inc.
208. Janis IL and Mann L: Decision making, New York, 1977, The Free Press.
209. Jarrard MM and Freeman JB: The effects of antibiotic ointments and antiseptics on the skin flora beneath subclavian catheter dressings during intravenous hyperalimentation J Surg Res 22:521-526, 1976.
210. Jarrard MM, Olson CM, and Freeman JB: Daily dressing change effects on skin flora beneath subclavian catheter dressings during total parenteral nutrition, J Parenteral Enteral Nutr 4:391-392, 1980.
211. Johnson J: Altering patients' response to surgery: an extension and replication, Res Nurs Health 1:111-121, 1978.
212. Johnson-Saylor MT, Pohl J, and Lowe-Wickson B: An assessment form for determining patients' health status and coping responses, Top Clin Nurs, pp 20-32, July 1982.
213. Jones SL: Family therapy. In Lezo S, ed: The American handbook of psychiatric nursing, Philadelphia, 1984, JB Lippincott Co.
214. Junginger J and Frame CI: Self report of the frequency and phenomenology of verbal hallucinations, J Nerv Ment Dis 173(3):149-155, 1985.

215. Kaminsky A and Molitor M: Validation study of the nursing diagnosis: decreased cardiac output. In McLane AM, ed: Classification of nursing diagnoses: proceedings of the Seventh Conference, St Louis, 1987, The CV Mosby Co.
216. Kao Lo CH and Kim MJ: Construct validity of sleep pattern disturbance: a methodological approach. In Hurley ME, ed: Classification of nursing diagnoses: proceedings of the Sixth Conference, St Louis, 1986, The CV Mosby Co.
217. Kaplan HS: The evaluation of sexual disorders, New York, 1983, Brunner/Mazel, Inc.
218. Kar SB, Schnitz M, and Dyer D: A psychosocial model of health behavior: implications for nutrition education, research and policy, Health Value 7:29-37, 1983.
219. Katz S: Index of independence in activities of daily living (Index of ADL). In Instruments for measuring nursing practice and other health care variables, vol 1, DHEW Pub No HRA 78.53, Washington, DC, 1981, US Government Printing Office.
220. Kavanaugh TB and Shepard RJ: Sexual activity after myocardial infarction, Can Med Assoc J 116:1250-1253, 1977.
221. Keenan CC: Loss of mobility, In Infante MS, ed: Crisis theory: a framework for nursing practice, Reston, Va, 1982, Reston Publishing Co.
222. Kenney RL: Decision analysis: an overview, Operations Res 30:803-838, 1982.
223. Kerfoot KM and Buckwalter KC: Sexual counseling. In Bulechek GM and McCloskey JC, eds: Nursing interventions: treatments for nursing diagnoses, Philadelphia, 1985, WB Saunders Co.
224. Kermani EJ: Violent psychiatric patients: a study, Am J Psychother 35(2):215-225, 1981.
225. Kim MJ, McFarland GK, and McLane AM: Pocket guide to nursing diagnoses, St Louis, 1984, The CV Mosby Co.
226. Kinney AB and Blount M: Effect of cranberry juice on urinary pH, Nurs Res 28:287-290, 1979.
227. Kinney AB, Blount M, and Dowell M: Urethral catheterization: pros and cons of an invasive but sometimes essential procedure, Geriatr Nurs 1:258-263, Dec 1980.
228. Kitabchi AE, Matteri R, and Murphy MB: Insulin delivery in DKA and HHNC, Diabetes Care 5(1):85-86, May-June 1982.
229. Knafl KA and Grace HK: Families across the life cycle: studies for nursing, Boston, 1978, Little, Brown & Co, Inc.
230. Kobashi-Schoot JAM, Hanewald GJFP, Van Dam FSAM, and Bruning PF: Assessment of malaise in cancer patients treated with chemotherapy, Cancer Nurs 8(6):306-378, 1985.
231. Konstantinides NN and Shronts E: Managing the basics, Am J Nurs 1312-1326, 1983.
232. Kunst-Wilson W and Cronenevett L: Nursing care for the emerging family: promoting parental behavior, Res Nurs Health 4:201-211, 1981.

233. Lamb MA: The sleeping patterns of patients with malignant and nonmalignant diseases, Cancer Nurs 5(5):389-396, 1982.
234. Lambert C and Lambert V: Psychosocial impacts created by chronic illness, Nurs Clin North Am 22(3):527, 1987.
235. Lancaster J: Adult psychiatric nursing, New York, 1980, Medical Examination Publishing Co, Inc.
236. Lapinski ML: Cardiovascular drugs and the elderly population, Heart Lung 11(5):430-433, 1982.
237. Larkin J: Factors influencing one's ability to adapt to chronic illness, Nurs Clin North Am 22(3):535-542, 1987.
238. Larsen GI: Chewing and swallowing. In Martin N, Holt NB, and Hicks DB, eds: Comprehensive rehabilitative nursing, New York, 1981, McGraw-Hill Book Co.
239. Larson M and Kim MJ: Respiratory muscle training with the incentive spirometer resistive breathing device, Heart Lung 13:341-345, 1984.
240. Lawrence PA: Home care for ventilator-dependent children: providing a chance to live a normal life, Dimens Crit Care Nurs 3(1):42-52, 1984.
241. Lazare A: Unresolved grief. In Lazare A, ed: Outpatient psychiatry diagnosis and treatment, Baltimore, 1979, Williams & Wilkins.
242. Lazarus RS: The costs and benefits of denial. In Breznita S, ed: The denial of stress, New York, 1983, International Universities Press, Inc.
243. Lazarus RS and Folkman S: Stress, appraisal and coping, New York, 1986, Springer Publishing Co, Inc.
244. Lean GR and Chamberlain K: Comparison of daily eating habits and emotional status of overweight persons successful or unsuccessful in maintaining a weight loss, J Consult Clin Psychol 61:108-115, 1973.
245. Ledray LE: A nursing developed model for the treatment of rape victims. In From accommodation to self-determination: nursing's role in the development of health care policy, Kansas City, Mo, 1982, American Academy of Nursing.
246. Lee BY et al: Topical application of povidone-iodine in the management of decubitus and stasis ulcers, J Am Geriatr Soc 27:306-307, July 1979.
247. Lego S, ed: The American handbook of psychiatric nursing, Philadelphia, 1984, JB Lippincott Co.
248. Leigh RJ and Turnberg LA: Fecal incontinence: the unvoiced symptom, Lancet 1349-1351, June 1982.
249. Lentz M: Selected aspects of deconditioning second to immobilization, Nurs Clin North Am 16(4):729-737, 1981.
250. Leske JS: Hyperglycemic hyperosmolar nonketotic coma: a nursing care plan, Crit Care Nurs 5(5):49-56, 1985.
251. Lester D: Southern subculture, personal violence (suicide and homicide), and firearms, Omega 17(2):183-186, 1986-1987.

252. Levitt EE: The psychology of anxiety, Hillsdale, NJ, 1980, Lawrence Erlbaum Associates, Inc.
253. Liberman RP, Kuehnel TG, Phipps CC, et al: Resource book for the mentally ill, Los Angeles, 1985, University of California Press.
254. Liberman RP, Massel HK, Mosk MD, and Wong SE: Social skills training for chronic mental patients, Hosp Community Psychiatry 36(4):396-403, 1985.
255. Liberman RP and Phipps CC: Innovative treatment and rehabilitation techniques for the chronic mentally ill. In Menninger WW and Hannah GT: The chronic mental patient, Washington, DC, 1987, American Psychiatric Press.
256. Lichentstein VR: The battered woman: guideline for effective nursing intervention, Issues Ment Health Nurs 3(3):237-250, 1981.
257. Lindan R, Joiner E, Freehafer AA, and Hazel C: Incidence and clinical features of autonomic dysreflexia in patients with spinal cord injury, Paraplegia 18:285-292, 1980.
258. Lingner C, Rolstad BS, Wetherill K, and Danielson S: Clinical trial of a moisture vapor-permeable dressing on superficial pressure sores, J Enterostomal Ther 11(4):147-149, 1984.
259. Linn D and Linn M: Healing life's hurts, Ramsey, NJ, 1978, Paulist Press.
260. Linn D, Linn M, and Fabricant S: Prayer course for healing life's hurts, Ramsey, NJ, 1983, Paulist Press.
261. Lion EM: Human sexuality in nursing process, New York, 1985, John Wiley & Sons, Inc.
262. Long BC and Phipps WJ: Essentials of medical-surgical nursing: a nursing process approach, St Louis, 1985, The CV Mosby Co.
263. Lorin MI: Elevated body temperature: symptomatic treatment, Consultant 20:130-131, 1980.
264. Luce J, Tyler M, and Pierson D: Therapy to improve airway clearance. In Luce J, Tyler M, and Pierson D, eds: Intensive respiratory care, Philadelphia, 1984, WB Saunders Co.
265. Luckmann J, Cowan M, and Pittman R: Nursing patients experiencing disturbances of peripheral vascular function. In Luckmann J and Sorensen KC eds: Medical-surgical nursing: a psychophysiologic approach, Philadelphia, 1974, WB Saunders Co.
266. Luckmann J and Sorensen K: Medical-surgical nursing, Philadelphia, 1980, WB Saunders Co.
267. Ludwig AM: Principles of clinical psychiatry, New York, 1980, Free Press.
268. MacLeod JH: Biofeedback in the management of partial anal incontinence, Dis Colon Rectum 26:244-246, 1983.
269. Maier G, Staua L, Morrow B, Van Rybroek G, and Bauman K: A model for understanding and managing cycles of aggression among psychiatric patients, Hosp Community Psychiatry 38:520-524, 1987.
270. Mandelstam D: Special techniques: strengthening pelvic floor muscles, Geriatr Nurs 1:251-252, 1980.

271. Manderino M and Bzdek V: Social skill building with chronic patients, J Psychosoc Nurs Ment Health Serv 25(9):18-23, 1987.
272. Margo A, Hemsley DR, and Slade PD: The effects of varying auditory input on schizophrenic hallucinations, Br J Psychiatry 139:122-127, 1981.
273. Marini JJ, Tyler ML, Hudson LD, Davis BS, and Huesby JS: Influence of head dependent positions on lung volume and oxygen saturation in chronic airflow obstruction, Am Rev Respir Dis 129:101-105, 1984.
274. Martin N, Holt NB, and Hicks D: Comprehensive rehabilitative nursing, New York, 1981, McGraw-Hill Book Co.
275. Maslow A: Towards a psychology of being, ed 2, New York, 1968, D Van Nostrand Co.
276. Matz A: Hypothermia: mechanisms and counter measures, Hosp Pract 21(1A):45-71, 1986.
277. Maxwell MH and Kleeman CR, eds: Clinical disorders of fluid and electrolyte metabolism, ed 3, San Francisco, 1980, McGraw-Hill Book Co.
278. May HJ, Gazda GM, Powell M, and Hauser G: Life skill training: psychoeducational training as mental health treatment, J Clin Psychol 41(3):359-367, 1985.
279. McCaffery M: Nursing management of the patient with pain, ed 2, Philadelphia, 1979, JB Lippincott Co.
280. McCarthy PA: Fetal alcohol syndrome and other alcohol-related birth defects, Nurs Pract 8(1):33-37, 1983.
281. McCaul KD: Sensory information, fear level, and reactions to pain, J Pers 48(4):494-504, 1980.
282. McCauley K and Weavery TE: Cardiac and pulmonary diseases: nutritional implications, Nurs Clin North Am 18:81-95, 1983.
283. McCorkle R and Young K: Development of a symptom distress scale, Cancer Nurs, pp 373-378, Oct 1978.
284. McCormick K and Burgio KL: Incontinence: update on nursing care measures, J Gerontol Nurs 10:16-23, 1984.
285. McCormick KA, Scheve AAS, and Leahy E: Nursing management of urinary incontinence in geriatric patients, Nurs Clin North Am 23(1):231-263, 1988.
286. McCourt AE: The measurement of functional deficit in quality assurance, Quality Assurance Update 5(3):1-3, 1981.
287. McCubbin H and Patterson J, eds: Systematic assessment of family stress, resources and coping, St Paul, 1981, University of Minnesota.
288. McFarland GK and McCann J: Self-perception—self-concept. In Thompson JM, McFarland GK, Hirsch JE, Tucker SM, and Bowers AC, eds: Clinical nursing, St Louis, 1986, The CV Mosby Co.
289. McFarland GK and Naschinski C: Impaired communication: a descriptive study, Nurs Clin North Am 20(4):775-785, 1985.
290. McFarland GK and Naschinski C: Communication. In Thompson JM, McFarland GK, Hirsch JE, Tucker SM, and Bowers AC,

eds: Clinical nursing, St Louis, 1986, The CV Mosby Co.

291. McFarland GK and Wasli EL: Nursing care of patients with psychiatric-mental health problems, grieving: dysfunctional, potential dysfunctional. In Kim MJ, McFarland GK, and McLane AM, eds: Pocket guide to nursing diagnosis, St Louis, 1984, The CV Mosby Co.
292. McFarland GK and Wasli EL: Coping-stress-tolerance. In Thompson JM, McFarland GK, Hirsch JE, Tucker SM, and Bowers AC, eds: Clinical nursing, St Louis, 1986, The CV Mosby Co.
293. McFarland GK and Wasli EL: Nursing diagnoses and process in psychiatric mental health nursing, Philadelphia, 1986, JB Lippincott Co.
294. McGee R: Hope: a factor influencing crisis resolution, Adv Nurs Sci 6(4):34-44, 1984.
295. McGlashan R: Strategies for rebuilding self-esteem in the cardiac patient, Dimens Crit Care Nurs, 1988.
296. McGuire TJ and Kramer VN: Autonomic dysreflexia in the spinal cord-injured: what the physician should know about this medical emergency, Postgrad Med 80(2):81-89, 1986.
297. McKay M, Davis M, and Famming P: Thoughts and feelings: the art of cognitive stress intervention, Richmond, Calif, 1981, New Harbinger Publications.
298. McLane AM, Krop H, and Mehta J: Psychosexual adjustment and counseling after myocardial infarction, Ann Intern Med 92(4):514-519, 1980.
299. McLane AM and McShane RE: Elimination. In Thompson JM, McFarland GK, Hirsch JE, Tucker SM, and Bowers AC, eds: Clinical nursing, St Louis, 1986, The CV Mosby Co.
300. McLane AM and McShane RE: Empirical validation of defining characteristics of constipation: a study of bowel elimination practices of healthy adults. In Hurley M, ed: Classification of nursing diagnoses: proceedings of the Sixth Conference, St Louis, 1986, The CV Mosby Co.
301. McLane AM and McShane RE: Constipation: proposed models for practice and research. In Maas M and Buckwalter KC, eds: Nursing diagnoses and intervention for the elderly, Menlo Park, Calif, Addison-Wesley Publishing Co, Inc (in press).
302. McLane AM, McShane RE, and Sliefert M: Constipation: conceptual categories of diagnostic indicators. In Kim MJ, McFarland GK, and McLane AM, eds: Classification of nursing diagnoses: proceedings of the Fifth National Conference, St Louis, 1984, The CV Mosby Co.
303. McShane RE and McLane AM: Constipation: consensual and empirical validation, Nurs Clin North Am 20:801-808, 1985.
304. McShane RE and McLane AM: Constipation: impact of etiological factors, J Gerontol Nurs 14(4):31-34, 1988.
305. Meinhart NT and McCaffery M: Pain: a nursing approach to

assessment and analysis, Norwalk, Conn, 1983, Appleton-Century-Crofts.

306. Meisenhelder JB: Self-esteem in women: the influence of employment and perception of husband's appraisals, Image 18:8-14, 1986.
307. Melzack R: The McGill pain questionnaire: major properties and scoring methods, Pain 1:277-299, 1975.
308. Menaghan EG: Individual coping efforts and family studies: conceptual and methodological issues. In McCubbin HI, Sussman MB, and Patterson JM, eds: Social stress and the family: advances and developments in family stress theory and research, New York, 1983, The Haworth Press, Inc.
309. Mercer RT: A theoretical framework for studying the factors that impact on the maternal role, Nurs Res 30:73-77, 1980.
310. Merenstein G and Gardner S: Handbook of neonatal intensive care, St Louis, 1985, The CV Mosby Co.
311. Merskey H: Development of a universal language of pain syndromes. In Bonica JJ et al, eds: Advances in pain research and therapy, vol 5, New York, 1978, Raven Press.
312. Metheny NA, Eisinberg P, and Spies M: Aspiration pneumonia in patients fed through nasoenteral tubes, Heart Lung 15(3):256-261, 1986.
313. Metheny NM, Snively WD, et al: Nurses' handbook of fluid balance, ed 4, Philadelphia, 1983, JB Lippincott Co.
314. Michael Reese Hospital and Medical Center: Nursing care plans: nursing diagnosis and intervention. In Gulanick M, Klopp A, and Galanes S, eds: St Louis, 1986, The CV Mosby Co.
315. Mickus D: Activities of daily living in women after myocardial infarction, Heart Lung 15:376-381, 1986.
316. Miller JF: Coping with chronic illness: overcoming powerlessness, Philadelphia, 1983, FA Davis Co.
317. Miller JF: Energy deficits in the chronically ill: the patient with arthritis. In Coping with chronic illness: overcoming powerlessness, Philadelphia, 1983, FA Davis Co.
318. Miller JF and Powers MJ: Development of an instrument to measure hope, Nurs Res 37:6-10, 1988.
319. Miller P, Wikoff RL, McMahon M, Garrett MJ, and Ringel K: Indicators of medical regimen adherence for myocardial infarction patients, Nurs Res 34:268-272, 1985.
320. Miller T, Wilson G, and Dumas M: Development and evaluation of social skills training for schizophrenic patients in remission, J Psychiatr Nurs Ment Health Serv 17:42-46, June 1979.
321. Minuchin S and Fishman HC: Family therapy techniques, Cambridge, 1981, Harvard University Press.
322. Moehrlin BA, Wolanin MO, and Burnside IM: Nutrition and the elderly. In Burnside IM, ed: Nursing and the aged, New York, 1981, McGraw-Hill Book Co.
323. Moen J, Chapman S, Sheehan A, and Carter P: Auxiliary versus

rectal temperatures in preterm infants under radiant warmers, JOGNN, pp 348-352, Sept-Oct 1987.
324. Molineux JB: Family therapy: a practical manual, Springfield, Ill, 1985, Charles C Thomas, Publisher.
325. Morgan JH: Behavioral treatment of obesity: the occupational health nurse's role, Occup Health Nurs 32:312-314, 1984.
326. Morse JM and Harrison MJ: Social coercion for weaning, J Nurse Midwife 32(4):205-210, 1987.
327. Morton P: Staff roles and responsibilities in incidents of patient violence, Arch Psychiatr Nurs 1:280-284, 1987.
328. Moss RC: Overcoming fear—a review of research on patient, family instruction, AORN J 43(5):1107-1114, 1986.
329. Mourad I: Nursing care of adults with orthopedic conditions, New York, 1980, John Wiley & Sons, Inc.
330. Moynihan BA and Duggan KC: The rape crisis team: consultation to critical care, Dimens Crit Care Nurs 1:354-359, 1982.
331. Mullin VI: Implementing the self-care concept in the acute care setting, Nurs Clin North Am 15(1):177-190, 1980.
332. Murphy GE: A conceptual framework for the choice of interventions in cognitive therapy, Cogn Ther Res 9(2):127-134, 1985.
333. Murray JF: Indications for mechanical aids to assist lung inflation in medical patients, Am Rev Respir Dis 122(5, part 2):121-125, 1980.
334. Neagley SR and Swillich CW: The influence of gastric filling and caloric consumption on the sensation of dyspnea in COPD, Am Rev Respir Dis 133(4, part 2, suppl.):A163, 1986.
335. Nehme AE and Trigger JA: Catheter dressings in central parenteral nutrition—a prospective randomized comparative study, Nutr Support Serv 4:42-50, 1984.
336. Neseman ME: Emergency care—tricks of the trade: hypothermia and hyperthermia, Consultant 25(13): 35-46, 1985.
337. Niederpruem MS: Autonomic dysreflexia, Rehabil Nurs 9:29-31, 1984.
338. Niedringhaus L: Hypovolemic shock. In Perry AG and Potter PA: Shock: comprehensive nursing management, St Louis, 1983, The CV Mosby Co.
339. North American Nursing Diagnosis Association: Classification of nursing diagnoses: proceedings of the Eighth Conference, Philadelphia, JB Lippincott Co (in press).
340. Norton C: Incontinence in the elderly. IV. Nursing the incontinent patient, Nurs Times Suppl 81(1):13-16, 1985.
341. Norton L and Comforti CG: The effects of body position on oxygenation, Heart Lung 14(1):45-51, 1985.
342. Nuernberger P: Freedom from stress: a holistic approach, Honesdale, Pa, 1981, The Himalayan International Institute of Yoga Science and Philosophy.
343. Nuwayhid K: Role function: theory and development. In Roy C: Introduction to nursing: an adaptation model, ed 2, Englewood Cliffs, NJ, 1984, Prentice-Hall.

344. Nyamathi A and Kashiwabara A: Preoperative anxiety—its effect on cognitive thinking, AORN J 47(1):164-170, 1988.
345. Olds SB, London ML, and Ladewig P: Maternal newborn nursing, ed 3, Menlo Park, Calif, 1988, Addison-Wesley Publishing Co, Inc.
346. Olson E, ed: The hazards of immobility, Am J Nurs 67(4):780-797, 1967.
347. O'Pray M: Working with families with infants with respiratory equipment in the home, Issues Compr Pediatr Nurs 10:113-121, 1987.
348. Ott CR, Sivarajan ES, Newton KM, Almes MJ, Bruce RA, Bergner M, and Gilson BS: A controlled randomized study of early cardiac rehabilitation: the Sickness Impact Profile as an assessment tool, Heart Lung 12:162-170, 1983.
349. Ouslander JG: Urinary incontinence in the elderly, West J Med 135:482-491, 1981.
350. Ozuna JM: A study of surgical patients' temperatures, Assoc OR Nurs J 28(2):240-245, 1978.
351. Pallet PJ and O'Brien MT: Nursing management of perceptual disturbances: textbook of neurological nursing, Boston, 1985, Little, Brown & Co, Inc.
352. Paloutzian R and Ellison C: Loneliness, spiritual well-being, and quality of life. In Peplau L and Perlman D, eds: Loneliness: a sourcebook of current theory, research, and therapy, New York, 1982, John Wiley & Sons, Inc.
353. Papadopoulous C, Beaumont C, Shelley SI, and Larrimore P: Myocardial infarction and sexual activity of the female patient, Arch Intern Med 143:1528, 1983.
354. Papp P: Setting the terms for therapy, Fam Ther Networker 8(1):42-47, 1984.
355. Pender NJ: Self-modification. In Bulechek GM and McCloskey J, eds: Nursing interventions: treatment for nursing diagnoses, Philadelphia, 1985, WB Saunders Co.
356. Pender NJ and Pender AR: Health promotion in nursing practice, ed 2, East Norwalk, Conn, 1987, Appleton & Lange.
357. Pentland B and Pennington CR: Acute diarrhea in the elderly, Age Aging 9:90-92, 1980.
358. Peplau H: Interpersonal relationships in nursing, New York, 1952, GP Putnam's Sons.
359. Peplau LA, Miceli M, and Morasch B: Loneliness and self-evaluation. In Peplau LA and Perlman D, eds: Loneliness, New York, 1982, John Wiley & Sons, Inc.
360. Peret KK and Stachowiak B: Alteration in health maintenance: conceptual base, etiology, and defining characteristics. In Kim MJ, McFarland GK, and McLane AM, eds: Classification of nursing diagnoses: proceedings of the Fifth National Conference, St Louis, 1984, The CV Mosby Co.
361. Pilch J: Wellness: your invitation to full life, Minneapolis, 1981, Winston Press.

362. Piper B: Fatigue. In Carriert V, Lindsey A, and West C, eds: Pathophysiological phenomena in nursing: human responses to illness, Philadelphia, 1986, WB Saunders Co.
363. Plaum S: Investigation of intake-output as a means of assessing body fluid balance, Heart Lung 8(3):495, 1979.
364. Pollman JW, Morris JJ, and Rose P: Is fiber the answer to constipation problems in the elderly? A review of literature, Int J Nurs Stud 15:107-114, 1978.
365. Pollock GH: The mourning liberation process in health and disease, Psychiatr Clin North Am 10(3):345-354, 1987.
366. Potempa K, Lopez M, Reid C, and Lawson L: Chronic fatigue, Image 18:165-169, 1986.
367. Powell C, Regan C, Fabri P, et al: Evaluation of Op-Site dressing for parenteral nutrition: a prospective, randomized study, J Parenteral Enteral Nutr 6:43, 1982.
368. Powell MF and Clayton MS: Efficacy of human relations training on selected coping behaviors of veterans in a psychiatric hospital, J Specialists Group Work 5:170-176, Aug 1980.
369. Preusser BA, Stone KS, Gonyon DS, Winningham ML, Groch KF, and Karl JE: Effects of two methods of preoxygenation on mean arterial pressure, cardiac output, peak airway pressure, and postsuctioning hypoxemia, Heart Lung 17(3):290-299, 1988.
370. Rainwater A and Christiansen K: Wellness/quality of life programs in a long-term care facility, Long Term Care Adm 12(4):13, 1984.
371. Raper AJ, Thompson WT, Shapiro W, and Patterson JG: Scalene and sternomastoid muscle function, J Appl Physiol 21:497-502, 1966.
372. Ravdin JI and Guerrant RL: Infectious diarrhea in the elderly, Geriatrics 38:95-101, 1983.
373. Reasoner RW: Self esteem through the life span, Fam Community Health 6:11-18, Aug 1983.
374. Redman BK: The process of patient education, ed 6, St Louis, 1988, The CV Mosby Co.
375. Reed-Ash C and Gianella A: Patient education, Cancer Nurs 5:261, 1982.
376. Rehm LP and Kaslow NJ: Behavioral approaches to depression: research results in clinical recommendations. In Franks CM, ed: New developments in behavior therapy: from research to clinical application, New York, 1984, The Haworth Press, Inc.
377. Reiss O and Oliveri M: Family paradigm and family coping: a proposal for linking the family's intrinsic adaptive capacities to its response to stress. In Kaslow FW, ed: The international book of family therapy, New York, 1982, Brunner/Mazel, Inc.
378. Remnet VL: The home assessment. In Burnside I, ed: Nursing and the aged, ed 2, New York, 1981, McGraw-Hill Book Co.
379. Richards KC and Bairnsfather BL: A description of night sleep patterns in the critical care unit, Heart Lung, 17(1):35-42, 1988.

380. Riddoch MJ and Humphreys GW: The effects of cueing on unilateral neglect, Neuropsychologia 21(6):589-599, 1983.
381. Ridgeway V and Mathews A: Psychological preparation for surgery: a comparison of methods, Br J Clin Psychol 21(4):271-280, 1982.
382. Robinson CH and Lawler MR: Normal and therapeutic nutrition, ed 16, New York, 1982, Macmillan Publishing Co.
383. Rogers CS, Morris S, and Taper LJ: Weaning from the breast: influences on maternal decisions, Pediatr Nurs 13(5):341-345, 1987.
384. Rombeau JL and Caldwell MD, eds: Enteral and tube feeding, Philadelphia, 1984, WB Saunders Co.
385. Rose MH and Thomas RB, eds: Children with chronic conditions: nursing in a family and community context, Orlando, Fla, Grune & Stratton, Inc.
386. Rothert ML and Talarczyk GJ: Patient compliance and the decision making process of clinicians and patients, J Compliance Health Care 2:55-71, 1987.
387. Rubenfeld MG: Diversional activity, deficit. In Thompson JM, McFarland GK, Hirsch JE, Tucker SM, and Bowers AC, eds: Clinical nursing, St Louis, 1986, The CV Mosby Co.
388. Rubenstein C, Shaver P, and Peplau LA: Loneliness, Hum Nature 58-65, Feb 1975.
389. Rush AJ, Beck AT, Kovacs M, Weissenburger J, and Hollon SD: Comparison of the effects of cognitive therapy and pharmacotherapy on hopelessness and self-concept, Am J Psychiatry 139(7):862-866, 1982.
390. Russel D: The measurement of loneliness. In Peplau LA and Perlman D, eds: Loneliness, New York, 1982, John Wiley & Sons, Inc.
391. Ryan P: Noncompliance. In Thompson JM, McFarland GK, Hirsch JE, Tucker SM, and Bowers AC, eds: Clinical nursing, St Louis, 1986, The CV Mosby Co.
392. Ryan P and Falco S: A pilot study to validate the etiologies and defining characteristics of the nursing diagnosis of noncompliance, Nurs Clin North Am 20(4):685-695, 1985.
393. Sanderson RG: The cardiac patient: a comprehensive approach, ed 2, Philadelphia, 1983, WB Saunders Co.
394. Saxton DF, Pelikan PK, Nugent PM, and Hyland PA: The Addison-Wesley manual for nursing practice, Menlow Park, Calif, 1983, Addison-Wesley Publishing Co.
395. Schacter FF: Sibling deidentification in the clinic: devil vs. angel, Fam Process 24(3):415-427, 1985.
396. Schauss A: Diet, crime, and delinquency, Berkeley, Calif, 1981, Parker Publishing Co.
397. Schmidt C: Withdrawal behavior of schizophrenics: application of Roy's Model, J Psychiatr Nurs Ment Health Serv 19:26-33, Nov. 1981.

398. Schroeder P and Gunta K: Comfort, alteration in: pain. In Thompson JM, McFarland GK, Hirch JE, Tucker SM, and Bowers AC, eds: Clinical nursing, St Louis, 1986, The CV Mosby Co.
399. Schultz J and Dark S: Manual of psychiatric nursing care plans, ed 2, Boston, 1986, Little, Brown & Co, Inc.
400. Schwartz-Fulton J, Colley R, Valanis B, et al: Hyperalimentation dressings and skin flora, Nat Intraven Ther Assoc 4:354, 1981.
401. Scrimshaw SC, Engle PL, Arnold L, and Haynes K: Factors affecting breastfeeding among women of Mexican origin or descent in Los Angeles, Am J Public Health 77(4):467-470, 1987.
402. Segal L: Brief family therapy. In Horne AM and Ohlsen MM, eds: Family counseling and therapy, Itasca, Ill, 1982, FE Peacock Publishers, Inc.
403. Sexton DL: The patient with peripheral arterial occlusive disease, Nurs Clin North Am 12:89-100, 1977.
404. Shah D et al: Cardiac output and pulmonary wedge pressure, Arch Surg 112:1161, 1977.
405. Sharp JT, Goldberg NB, Druz WS, Fishman HC, and Danon J: Thoracoabdominal motion in chronic obstructive pulmonary disease, Am Rev Respir Dis 115:47-56, 1977.
406. Shekleton ME and Nield M: Ineffective airway clearance related to artificial airway, Nurs Clin North Am 22(1):167-178, 1987.
407. Shelp EE and Perl M: Denial in clinical medicine: a reexamination of the concept and its significance, Arch Intern Med 145:697-699, 1985.
408. Shepard AM, Blannin JP, and Fineley RCL: Changing attitudes in the management of urinary incontinence: the need for specialist nursing, Br Med J 284:645-646, 1982.
409. Shepard AM, Tribe E, and Tarrens MJ: Simple practical techniques in the management of urinary incontinence, Int Rehabil Med 4:15-19, 1982.
410. Sideleau BF: Irrational beliefs and interventions, J Psychosoc Nurs Ment Health Serv 25(3):18-24, 1987.
411. Simmons N: Disorders in oral speech and language function. In Unphred I, ed: Neurological rehabilitation, St Louis, 1985, The CV Mosby Co.
412. Simons AD, Garfield SL, and Murphy GE: The process of change in cognitive therapy and pharmacotherapy for depression, Arch Gen Psychiatry 41(1):45-51, 1984.
413. Simons AD et al: Cognitive therapy and pharmacotherapy for depression, Arch Gen Psychiatry 43(1):43-48, 1986.
414. Simonson G: Caring for the patient with acute myelocytic leukemia, Am J Nurs 3:304-309, 1988.
415. Skinner JS: Sexual relations and the cardiac patient. In Pollack ML and Schmidt DC, eds: Heart disease and rehabilitation, ed 2, New York, 1986, John Wiley & Sons, Inc.
416. Slade PD: The external control of auditory hallucinations: an information theory analysis, Br J Soc Clin Psychol 13:73-79, 1974.
417. Slimmer LW and Brown RT: Parent's decision making process in

medication administration for control of hyperactivity, J School Health 55:221-225, 1985.

418. Smith B and Cantrell P: Distance in nurse-patient encounters, J Psychosoc Nurs Ment Health Serv 22(2):22-26, 1988.
419. Smith M: Duration experience for bed confined subjects: a replication-refinement, Nurs Res 28(3):139-144, 1979.
420. Sneed DS: Hyperosmolar hyperglycemic nonketotic coma, Crit Care Q 3(2):29-44, 1980.
421. Snyder M: Independent nursing interventions, New York, 1985, John Wiley & Sons, Inc.
422. Snyder-Halpern R and Verran JA: Instrumentation to describe subjective sleep characteristics in healthy subjects—Verran & Snyder-Halpern (VSH) sleep scale, Res Nurs Health 10(3):155-163, 1987.
423. Speer JJ and Sachs B: Selecting the appropriate family assessment tool, Pediatr Nurs 11:349-355, 1985.
424. Spielman AJ, Saskin P, and Thorpy MJ: Treatment of chronic insomnia by restriction of time in bed, Sleep 10(1):45-56, 1987.
425. Spittell JA: Recognition and management of chronic atherosclerotic occlusive peripheral arterial disease, Mod Concepts Cardiovasc Dis 50(4):19-23, 1981.
426. Stafford MJ: Nursing care of patients with cardiovascular problems, cardiac output, alteration in, decreased. In Kim MJ, McFarland GK, and McLane AM, eds: Pocket guide to nursing diagnoses, St Louis, 1984, The CV Mosby Co.
427. Steckel SB: Patient contracting, Norwalk, Conn, 1982, Appleton-Century-Crofts.
428. Stewart M: Measurement of clinical pain. In Jacox A, ed: Pain: a source book for nurses and other health professionals, Boston, 1977, Little, Brown & Co., Inc.
429. Stewart T and Shields CR: Grief in chronic illness: assessment and management, Arch Phys Med Rehabil 66:447-450, 1985.
430. Stinemetz, Jinney, et al: Rx for stress: a nurses' guide, Palo Alto, Calif, 1984, Bull Publishing Co.
431. Stoner C: Learned helplessness: analysis and application, Oncol Nurs Forum 12(11):31-35, 1985.
432. Strandness DE: Vascular diseases of the extremities. In Isselbacher K et al, eds: Harrison's principles of internal medicine, ed 9, New York, 1980, McGraw-Hill Book Co.
433. Streff MB: Examining family growth and development: a theoretical model, Adv Nurs Sci 3(4):61-69, 1981.
434. Stroot VR, Lee CA, and Barrett CA: Fluids and electrolytes: a practical approach, Philadelphia, 1984, FA Davis Co.
435. Tallis R: Incontinence in the elderly. II. Treating the impairment, Nurs Times 80(44):5-8, 1984.
436. Tallis R: Incontinence in the elderly. III. Preventing the disability, Nurs Times 80(48):9-12, 1984.
437. Tallis R and Norton C: Incontinence in the elderly. I. The rehabilitative approach, Nurs Times 80(39):1-4, 1984.

438. Tanberg D and Sklar D: Effect of tachypnea on the estimation of body temperature by an oral thermometer, N Engl J Med 308:945-956, 1983.
439. Teasdale K: The withdrawn schizophrenic, Nurs Times 82:32-34, Feb 1986.
440. Tennes K and Blackard C: Maternal alcohol consumption, birth weight, and minor physical anomalies, Am J Obstet Gynecol 138(7):774-780, 1980.
441. Thomas SA, Sappington E, Gross HS, Noctor M, Friedmann E, and Lynch JJ: Denial in coronary care patients—an objective reassessment, Heart Lung 12:74-80, 1983.
442. Thompson J: Injury, potential for. In Thompson JM, McFarland GK, Hirsch JE, Tucker SM, and Bowers AC, eds: Clinical nursing, St Louis, 1986, The CV Mosby Co.
443. Thompson JM, McFarland GK, Hirsch JE, Tucker SM, and Bowers AC, eds: Clinical nursing, St Louis, 1986, The CV Mosby Co.
444. Thompson WG and Heaton KW: Functional bowel disorders in apparently healthy people, Gastroenterology 79:283-288, 1980.
445. Tilton C and Maloof M: Diagnosing the problems in stroke, Am J Nurs 82:596-601, 1982.
446. Topf M and Dambacher B: Teaching interpersonal skills: a model for facilitating optimal interpersonal relations, J Psychiatr Nurs Ment Health Serv 19:29-33, Dec 1981.
447. Toth JC: The person with coronary artery disease and risk factors. In Guzzetta C and Dossey BM: Cardiovascular nursing: bodymind tapestry, St Louis, 1984, The CV Mosby Co.
448. Travis J and Ryan R: Wellness workbook: a guide to attaining high level wellness, Berkeley, Calif, 1986, Ten Speed Press.
449. Trelvar DM and Stechmiller J: Pulmonary aspiration in tube-fed patients with artificial airways, Heart Lung 13(6):667-671, 1984.
450. Tudhope M: Management of pressure ulcers with a hydrocolloid occlusive dressing: results in twenty-three patients, J Enterostomal Ther 11(3):102-105, 1984.
451. Tupin JP: The violent patient: a strategy for management and diagnosis, Hosp Community Psychiatry 34(1):37-40, 1983.
452. Turner J: Nursing intervention in patients with peripheral vascular disease, Nurs Clin North Am 21(2):233-240, 1986.
453. Twycross RG: Narcotic analgesics in clinical practice. In Bonica JJ et al, eds: Advances in pain research and therapy, vol 5, New York, 1983, Raven Press.
454. Tyler ML: Complications of positioning and chest physiotherapy, Respir Care 27:458-466, 1982.
455. Tyler ML: The respiratory effects of body positioning and immobilization, Respir Care 29(5):472-483, 1984.
456. Umbarger CC: Structural family therapy, New York, 1984, Grune & Stratton, Inc.
457. Underhill SL, Woods SL, Sivarajan ES, Halpenny CJ, et al: Cardiac nursing, Philadelphia, 1982, JB Lippincott Co.

458. Underwood BA: Evaluating the nutritional status of individuals: a critique of approaches, Nutr Rev Suppl: 213-223, May 1986.
459. Vale RJ: Normothermia: its place in operative and postoperative care, Anaesthesia 28(5):241-245, 1973.
460. Van Deusen J: Unilateral neglect, Am J Occup Ther 42(7):441-448, 1988.
461. Vander A, Sherman J, and Luciano D: Coordinated body functions: circulation. In Vander A, Sherman J, and Luciano D, eds: Human physiology: the mechanisms of body function, ed 2, New York, 1975. McGraw-Hill Book Co.
462. Vander A, Sherman J, and Luciano D: Regulation of organic metabolism and energy balance. In Vander A, Sherman J, and Luciano D, eds: Human physiology: the mechanisms of body function, ed 2, New York, 1975, McGraw-Hill Book Co.
463. Varricchio CG: Selecting a tool for measuring fatigue, Oncol Nurs Forum 12(4):122-127, 1985.
464. Ventura JN: Parent coping behaviors, parent functioning, and infant temperament and characteristics, Nurs Res 31:269-273, 1982.
465. Vogt G, Miller M, and Esluer M: Mosby's manual of neurological care, St Louis, 1985, The CV Mosby Co.
466. Voith AM: Alterations in urinary elimination concepts, research and practice, Rehabil Nurs 13(3):122-131, 1988.
467. Voith AM and Smith DA: Validation of the nursing diagnosis of urinary retention, Nurs Clin North Am 20:723-729, 1985.
468. Vuchinich S: Starting and stopping spontaneous family conflicts, J Marriage Fam 49(3):591-601, 1987.
469. Wabrek AJ and Burchell RC: Male sexual dysfunction associated with coronary heart disease, Arch Sex Behav 9:69-75, 1980.
470. Waldo MC, Roath M, Levine W, and Freedman R: A model to teach parenting skills to schizophrenic mothers, Hosp Community Psychiatry 38:1110-1112, 1987.
471. Walker M and Driscoll G, eds: Breast feeding your baby, ed 2, Wayne, NJ, 1981, Avery Publishing Group, Inc.
472. Warale J and Beinort H: Binge eating: a theoretical review, Br J Clin Psychol 20:97-109, 1981.
473. Warbinek E and Wyness MA: Designing nursing care for patients with peripheral arterial occlusive disease. I. Update, Cardiovasc Nurs 22(1):1-2, 1986.
474. Wasserman AL: A prospective study of the impact of home monitoring on the family, Pediatrics 74(3):323-329, 1984.
475. Watzlawick P: The language of change: elements of therapeutic communication, New York, 1978, Basic Books, Inc, Publishers.
476. Wehmer MA and Baldwin BJ: Inadvertent hypothermia, AORN J 44(5):788-796, 1986.
477. Weisman AD: On dying and denying, New York, 1982, Behavioral Publications.
478. Weitzman J: Engaging the severely dysfunctional family in treatment: basic considerations, Fam Process 24:473-485, 1985.

479. Welch D: Anticipatory grief reactions in family members of adult patients, Issues Ment Health Nurs 4:149-158, 1982.
480. Weldy NJ: Body fluids and electrolytes, a programmed presentation, St Louis, 1980, The CV Mosby Co.
481. Wenger NK and Hellerstein HK, eds: Rehabilitation in the coronary patient, ed 2, New York, 1984, John Wiley & Sons, Inc.
482. White JH: The process of embarking on a weight control program, Health Care Wom Int 5:77-91, 1984.
483. White JH and Schroeder MA: When your client has a weight problem: nursing assessment, Am J Nurs 81:550, 1981.
484. Whitney JD, Fellows BJ, and Larson E: Do mattresses make a difference? J Gerontol Nurs 10(9):20-25, 1984.
485. Wild L: Cardiovascular problems. In Carnevali D and Patrick M, eds: Nursing management for the elderly, ed 2, Philadelphia, 1986, JB Lippincott Co.
486. Wild L: Vascular structural disorders. In Patrick M, Woods S, Craven R, Rokosky J and Bruno P, eds: Medical-surgical nursing: pathophysiological concepts, Philadelphia, 1986, JB Lippincott Co.
487. Williams A: A study of factors contributing to skin breakdown, Nurs Res 21(3):238-243, 1972.
488. Wistrom D: Role playing, J Psychosoc Nurs 25(6):21-24, 1987.
489. Wolanin MO and Phillips LRF: Confusion: prevention and care, St Louis, 1981, The CV Mosby Co.
490. Woods N: Human sexuality in health and illness, ed 3, St Louis, 1984, The CV Mosby Co.
491. Worden JW: Grief-counseling and grief therapy, New York, 1982, Springer Publishing Co, Inc.
492. Wright PF, Thompson J, McKee KT Jr, Vaughn WK, Sell SH, and Karzon DT: Patterns of illness in the highly febrile young child: epidemiological, clinical, and laboratory correlates, Pediatrics 67:694-700, 1981.
493. Wyness MA: Perceptual dysfunction: nursing assessment and management, J Neurosurg Nurs 17(2):105-110, 1985.
494. Yocum CJ: The differentiation of fear and anxiety. In Kim MJ, McFarland GK, and McLane AM, eds: Classification of nursing diagnoses: proceedings of the Fifth National Conference, St Louis, 1984, The CV Mosby Co.
495. Yoder LE, Jones SL, and Jones PK: The association between health care behavior and attitudes, Health Values 9:24-31, 1985.
496. Yodufsky SC, Silver JM, Jackson W, Endicott J, and Williams D: The overt aggression scale for the objective rating of verbal and physical aggression, Am J Psychiatry 143(1)35-39, 1986.
497. Yodofsky SC, Stevens L, Silver J, Barsa J, and Williams D: Propranolol in the treatment of rage and violent behavior associated with Korsakoff's psychosis, Am J Psychiatry 141(1):114-115, 1984.
498. Young HF, Bentall RP, Slade PP, and Dewey ME: The role of brief instructions and suggestibility in the elicitation of auditory

and visual hallucinations in normal and psychiatric subjects, J Nerv Ment Dis 175(1):41-48, 1987.

499. Zell SC and Kurtz KJ: Severe exposure hypothermia: a resuscitation protocol, Ann Emergency Med 14:339, April 1985.
500. Ziegler CC: Systemic lupus erythematosus and systemic sclerosis, Nurs Clin North Am 19:673-695, 1984.

BIBLIOGRAPHY

NANDA proceedings

Gebbie KM and Lavin MA, eds: Classification of nursing diagnoses: proceedings of the First National Conference, St Louis, 1975, The CV Mosby Co.

Gebbie KM, ed: Classification of nursing diagnoses: summary of the Second National Conference, St Louis, 1976, Clearinghouse.

Kim MJ and Moritz DA, eds: Classification of nursing diagnoses: proceedings of the Third and Fourth National Conferences, St Louis, 1982, McGraw-Hill Book Co.

Kim MJ, McFarland GK, and McLane AM, eds: Classification of nursing diagnoses: proceedings of the Fifth National Conference, St Louis, 1984, The CV Mosby Co.

Hurley ME, ed: Classification of nursing diagnoses: proceedings of the Sixth Conference, St Louis, 1986, The CV Mosby Co.

McLane A, ed: Classification of nursing diagnoses: proceedings of the Seventh Conference, St Louis, 1987, The CV Mosby Co.

POCKET GUIDE

(in native languages, alphabetically)

CHINESE Kim MJ, McFarland GK, and McLane AM, eds: Huli chentuan shouts'e (Pocket guide to nursing diagnoses), translated by Ts'ai Hsin-Ling, Taiwan, 1986, Huahsing Publishing Co., Ltd.

ENGLISH Kim MJ, McFarland GK, and McLane AM, eds: Pocket guide to nursing diagnosis, St Louis, 1984, The CV Mosby Co.

FRENCH Kim MJ, McFarland GK, and McLane AM, eds: Guide pratique des diagnostics infirmiers, Quebec, Canada, 1985, Gaêtan Morin.

SPANISH Kim MJ, McFarland GK, and McLane AM, eds: Diagnostico en enfermeria, Madrid, 1986, Interamericana.

NOTES

NOTES

NOTES

NOTES

NOTES

NOTES

NOTES

NOTES

INDEX

Italic entries indicate corresponding nursing care plans.